AUTOPATHY: A HOMEOPATHIC JOURNEY TO HARMONY
Healing and Self-Healing with Water and Saliva

Jiri Cehovsky

Autopathy:
A Homeopathic Journey
to Harmony

Healing and Self-Healing
with Water and Saliva

www.autopathy.info

Autopathy: A Homeopathic Journey to Harmony
Healing and Self-Healing with Water and Saliva
Second revised edition
Translated by William Thomas McEnchroe MA (Oxon)
Edited by Nick Churchill MA(Oxon), RSHom
© Jiri Cehovsky, 2003, 2006
ISBN 80–86936–03–1
Alternativa Publishing Ltd.
Kosikarska 667, 156 00 Prague 5
Czech Republic, European Union
info@alternativa.cz
www.autopathy.info

Contents

Author's Foreword

Autopathy is a holistic method. Its roots stretch deep into the past and it has emerged gradually through the wisdom of generations. Although references to autopathic approaches can be found in homeopathic, ayurvedic and other literature, this is the first systematic exposition of the method. It contains my personal observations, which, although recorded over a period of only four years, are supported by more than twenty-two years of experience in treating people through classical homeopathy. Autopathy is thus a nascent method. We are just beginning to learn the laws behind the holistic effects of using our own, homeopathically highly-diluted saliva or other secretions. The book does not contain a set of instructions on how to act in specific situations, but rather a record of my experience, limited as this is by time and other factors. Autopathy should not be a substitute for homeopathy or other alternative or conventional and specialised methods of treatment. It should be a further contribution, another approach to holistic healing, offering new and—my experience permits me to say—as yet unimagined opportunities. It stems from an understanding that is shared by certain religious systems, one of which is Buddhism: that everyone carries their cure within themselves.

Part I.
ORIGINS

1. A Case History

Vaclav first came to my homeopathic consulting room in the spring of 2002. He was thirty-five, thin, with a scabrous face covered in large, red, and in places, suppurating sores. He showed me the same condition on his chest and all over his arms, shoulders and back. The atopic eczema itched and forced him to scratch the affected areas. The intense, unpleasant, painful and unrelenting sensations sometimes caused him to suffer from fevers accompanied by shivering. He told me that it was liable to deteriorate at any time, including in response to the slightest psychological stress. Doctors had treated his illness since early childhood. After puberty he had lived for several years without atopic eczema, although he had suffered badly from hay fever. From the age of twenty-seven, however, he had again been forced to start visiting dermatological clinics.

In recent years he had also begun to suffer pain at the base of his right ribcage. This had been diagnosed by doctors as a poorly-functioning gallbladder. The pains became more frequent, particularly after eating garlic, fatty foods or after overeating. Occasionally, he suffered serious episodes that forced him to withdraw temporarily from everyday life. He had suffered such an episode just three days before visiting me. The episodes were characterised by stomach cramp, pain throughout the abdomen, flatulence and diarrhoea and a raised temperature: 37.6⁰C during his most recent episode.

Vaclav was seriously concerned that if his medical condition were to continue to deteriorate at the same rate things could end badly. This was why he had decided to pursue a holistic approach to treatment; three months earlier he had registered with me and now he had come in the hope that I would succeed smoothly and swiftly where all my predecessors had failed.

At first, his case didn't seem particularly suited to homeopathic treatment as the pathological and psychological profile didn't provide any reliable indication of a remedy (I will provide a brief explanation later). I had only just begun to practise autopathy and was only using it to treat a few chronically-ill patients (although partly based on previous treatments, as I will explain later). I therefore hesitated somewhat before recommending autopathy. I told him that with homeopathy, which I had been practising for twenty-two years, we look for a natural substance that can resonate with the patient's whole personality and re-tune his organism into a state of health. The substance must always be strongly diluted, down to intangibly small "amounts". For some it might be cat's milk (*Lac felinum*), for another triturated bee (*Apis mellifica*), while others resonate with snake poison (*Lachesis*) and still others with human disease products (*Medorrhinum, Psorinum*)—obviously infinitesimally diluted and therefore harmless—with the plant *Lycopodium*, or with minerals such as sulphur or phosphorus. To find the right substance can sometimes be complicated and professionally very demanding. The closer the substance is in character to the patient, the more striking the resonance and the more effective the treatment, and the deeper and longer-lasting the cure. The task is to find the right remedy for the patient as quickly as possible. With homeopathy we seek a substance that is tuned as closely as possible to the patient. In autopathy, however, we don't use substances taken from surrounding nature, such as plants, or from the bodies of animals or people. Instead, autopathy advocates using a substance from the patient's own body—saliva, a substance that holds the same vibrational pattern as the patient, but of course in a different state to that found in the mouth. Water is used to dilute it to a fine-matter level (from a materialistic point of view, a non-material level) analogous to the method used in homeopathy, and then it is used just once. The infinitesimally-diluted saliva carries all the information about the organism, its vibrational imprint, and guarantees full resonance of the fine-matter vibrational organising principle that everyone has inside them. I gave Vaclav a special glass bottle (later I called it an "Autopathic Bottle") and instructions on how to prepare the autopathic substance at home to a high potency (I will explain in detail later). I told him: "In simple terms, just spit into the glass, pour in normal table water or distilled water and after it has been diluted pour a few drops onto your tongue. Throw the glass away and come back in a few weeks for a follow-up." Having finished, and finding it difficult to conceal my curiosity, I looked into his intelligent and suffering face and waited to see how he would react to a proposal that might have come from the realms of science fiction (or detective fiction if it had involved fraud). To my surprise, he didn't even blink an eye. "Fine," he said. His trust perhaps stemmed partly from the fact that he had seen me half a year earlier on a television programme devoted to health matters where I had appeared with the daughter of a children's doctor whom I had once cured of a similar eczema condition using homeopathy. He took away with him the Autopathic Bottle and the printed instructions on how to prepare the autopathic preparation at home in the bathroom.

He rang me two weeks later. He told me that he could still feel his gallbladder but that he had experienced no further episodes or pronounced pain. The first week after using the autopathic preparation the eczema had worsened somewhat; in the second week it began to disappear from his face, leaving instead some protuberances on the skin that looked like pimples. Now, two weeks after applying the treatment, there was almost nothing on his face.

We met again three months after he had taken the single autopathic preparation. He took out the notes in which I had advised him to record significant changes in the state of his health so that he could refer to them at the follow-up. As before, he agreed that I should record the examination on video (I sometimes use video tapes for my lectures at the Homeopathic Academy). The video was remarkable, despite the fact that his face was now rather uninteresting and completely normal—that is, without eczema and without scabs. He reported that the eczema had disappeared everywhere with the exception of a mild rash on the crooks of his elbows. All feelings of pain had disappeared as well. It had taken only six weeks following the application of the autopathic preparation to arrive at this state. The gallbladder was much improved and no longer gave him pain. He had suffered no crises from his gallbladder throughout this period and only "knew" about the gallbladder when he erred in his diet. In general he felt very well and healthy, which for him was a completely new feeling in life. We parted agreeing that he would contact me if any complications occurred.

Two and a half years after using the autopathic preparation, which was repeated once, and after several further follow-ups, he is entirely free of any ailments and moreover does not even follow a diet.

This is only one of many cases I have experienced where so-called "incurable" chronic illnesses have been overcome with the harmonizing effect of autopathy. In this instance the treatment was incredibly uncomplicated. I should point out at the beginning that the process is not always so rapid or so straightforward.

2. How My Eyes Were Opened

When we encounter something new and unfamiliar we always ask questions. How was it possible that Vaclav could have been helped by a diluted version of his own saliva? Especially when even the word "diluted" is an understatement. In this case it was 10^{600}. It's known that at dilution levels of 10^{24} the so-called Avogadro limit is exceeded, which means that the "solution" can no longer contain any particle of the original substance. Not only that, but as the surprised mother of a small boy jokingly exclaimed when I proposed autopathic treatment using saliva: "How could diluted saliva help cure him when he's been swallowing the stuff undiluted all his life?"

I'll try to answer that as concisely as possible, but don't expect an answer that would fit on a telegram. Despite the surprising simplicity of its application, getting to the root of things is actually quite complicated. It has taken me twenty-two years to arrive at the stage described in this book. And because I share the opinion of many contemporary physicists that it is impossible to separate the observer from the process that he is observing, that entirely objective reports and research do not exist because the relationship between the researcher and the researched subject is one of constant interaction, I shall give a brief description of my own development in this field.

Up to the age of thirty I lived "like anyone else". This means that I didn't look after my health because I didn't consider it necessary. I blamed my problems on others, particularly the authorities, poor teachers, lack of money, the weather and so on. Every few years I would go to the health centre for penicillin for a sore throat. But all this changed at the age of thirty-three. It began with a high fever, which was subsequently aggravated by stomach pains. After taking antibiotics the fever passed but the pain in the stomach, or more precisely the lower abdomen, remained. Not only that but I began to have problems passing water. I visited a leading medical figure who gave me a rectal examination and said I had an inflamed prostate. I went on visiting him with no change in my symptoms for another year, diligently consumed my prescribed Biseptol and other delicacies and waited for the conventional medicines to take effect. This didn't happen and the doctor informed me after a year that I would have to get accustomed to the problems as they were of a chronic nature and I would never find a doctor who could relieve me of them. He was a decent, grey-haired main with a great deal of experience. I believed him. Then, in 1980, I threw myself into the study of works on herbal remedies. Some time later my sister, who lived in England, sent me homeopathic literature which, when piled up, measured around three quarters of a metre. Later she also sent me remedies. Another year went by and my complaints, which I had treated homeopathically using remedies that I found in weighty homeopathic books, disappeared, never to return over the following twenty-two years. This persuaded me that it is sometimes necessary to seek the truth elsewhere than in official institutions and school curricula. Thus began my homeopathic period, and it continues to this day. When I was thirty-three, few people in my circles even knew what homeopathy meant. I made it my mission to educate them and in the pub over a beer, or at the office where I was employed as an editor of children's publications, I would patiently explain the subject and examine friends and colleagues and supply them with homeopathic pills. One colleague had problems passing water: I gave him a solution I had diluted myself—potentised parsley—and it immediately passed. Another suffered from hay fever—after taking potentised kitchen salt it improved so much that he never again had to take conventional medicines. There were several such cases and all expressed their satisfaction. My small children no longer had to spend long hours at the doctor with bronchial and sinus problems. Whereas previously they had missed hundreds of hours of school, they now missed practically nothing. Sometimes we would even let them stay at home so they wouldn't feel bad about having to go to school far more often than the other children.

All this was made possible by potentised or highly-diluted plants, minerals and snake poisons. I produced many of the preparations myself. Homeopathy quite simply became my life and I became a homeopathic healer. A few years later I began to lecture and publish specialist homeopathic literature and diagnostic software, to invite teachers of homeopathy from England, India, Germany and Holland to lecture at my homeopathic schools, to publish a specialist homeopathic magazine and to work in the committee of the Homeopathic Medical Society which was established in the early nineteen hundreds. I understood that homeopathy represented a new value in the history of human culture. In addition to discovering homeopathy I had also found in Buddhist philosophy the explanation of certain fundamental questions that I had been asking. I also realised that both have striking similarities.

3. Fine-Matter Substances

The personal preparation of homeopathic potencies is an invaluable life experience. It opens up new space for reflection. At the pharmacy, homeopathic pills in glass or plastic bottles are virtually indistinguishable from other medicines. But when you come to prepare a homeopathic remedy yourself, following the same procedure as Samuel Hahnemann, who discovered homeopathy and the healing effect of highly-diluted substances, you will understand that you are practically on the same ground as alchemists, yogis and shamans: you are making good magic and producing Nothing from Something. After emptying and refilling the flask three times there is already nothing left of the original few drops of plant tincture, but you continue adding distilled water and each time continue to transfer one hundredth of the volume to another bottle, maybe thirty or sixty times. And the resulting preparation works and cures where other medications have failed. Not only that, but the preparation of the highly-diluted material is derived from a substance that in its original state has no effect on health whatsoever; for example gold or kitchen salt! The finer and more diluted the Something, the more effective it is. The less substance there is, the more it resembles thought—the strongest and most influential thing there is or ever has been. The substance loses its gross material form and is elevated to an ideal, fine-matter level, from where everything radiates "down" to the material world. And the further it falls the more it is devalued and the more remote it becomes from its ideal, "perfect" form. The higher it is, the closer it comes to perfection.

The term "fine-matter" comes from the Buddhist canon, in which it signifies higher levels of existence that cannot be attained by our earthly senses. Plato was one of those who remarked that the material world is merely the product, the reflection of the fine, immaterial world of the Idea. The same concepts are found in the Jewish Kabbalah, yoga, alchemy, Buddhism and the Bible, where reference is made to Paradise, a higher, subtle world from which Man was expelled as a result of his desires and wrongdoings to the gross, material world. This hierarchical system, which stretches from the subtle above to the material below, is well expressed in the shape of European church domes and Buddhist stupas. From the slender, light and often gilded summit above to the massive, corpulent base. The form of a pyramid testifies to the same process.

The idea of a higher, immaterial area which is the cause of gross material phenomena lies at the core of homeopathic philosophy. Hahnemann calls it spiritual, and it is analogous with "fine matter" in Buddhism. In paragraphs nine and ten of his *Organon*, the founding work of the discipline (see Bibliography), Hahnemann says that "In the state of health the spirit-like vital force (dynamis) animating the material human organism reigns in supreme sovereignty", and "Only because of the immaterial being (vital principle, vital force), that animates it in health and in disease can it feel and maintain its vital functions".

Hahnemann (1755–1843) was the younger contemporary of Emanuel Swedenborg (1688–1772) and was undoubtedly profoundly inspired by the ideas of the Swedish philosopher. The latter based his system on knowledge that he acquired in states of higher perception, in which he visited superior, heavenly worlds, conversed with angels and was instructed in how the universe worked, structured hierarchically from the gross material sphere to the most subtle heavenly realms—of which he recounted that there were several, hierarchically superior one to another. Swedenborg's description of the heavenly worlds closely resembles the reports of meditating Buddhist monks and yogis, who also visited higher fine-matter worlds or higher levels of reality. There are many similar descriptions in the Pali Buddhist canon recounting the stories of the Buddha and his disciples.

Swedenborg, who came from a Christian tradition (his father was a Protestant bishop and confessor to the Swedish queen), deserves extended mention here. Not only did he profoundly influence the development of European thought at the end of the eighteenth and beginning of the nineteenth centuries, he also stands at the philosophical origins of homeopathy and the production and use of highly-diluted, potentised substances.

One of Swedenborg's fundamental beliefs is that man is a multidimensional being who lives both in the gross material sphere on earth and, through his thought and feelings, in a higher sphere, in heaven. This higher, heavenly part of man he called the "Inner Man". Something must first happen in the fine-matter, heavenly sphere before it is manifested in the gross-matter, earthly sphere, in the body. These spheres are firmly connected and the lower sphere is continually, moment by moment, generated by its higher equivalent. Swedenborg wrote that not even "the smallest hair on an animal" can move without this event having its roots in the higher sphere. The origin of any phenomenon, thing or event is always fine matter, with the influence extending downwards to the gross material sphere. The fine-matter, heavenly sphere is not however external to man but on the contrary rests inside him. The journey upwards does not mean an outer but an inner journey. A similar path of thought had already been followed by the Sufis and in the Christian tradition the Rosicrucians, who likened man to a string, stretched and vibrating between heaven and earth. Consciousness can move upwards along this string to the more subtle vibrations or downwards to the lower, material vibrations. We will return to this image of a string later.

But for the moment let's continue with Swedenborg and in particular his followers among the ranks of homeopaths. The Americans Constantine Hering and James Tyler Kent were among the more important. Together with their pupils and families, both made regular visits to Swedenborg's temple of his New Church. Together, they were the authors of modern homeopathic philosophy and methods of treatment using highly-diluted substances, while essentially abiding by Swedenborg's view of the organisation of the universe. Kent wrote that man can be imagined as a point with around him three concentric circles. The point is the Inner Man, Man with a capital M, spiritual man who around him creates in the first circle the mind, in the second emotion and in the third the material physical organs. The organisation of the entire system emanates from the centre. Illness means interference to the organisation managed from the centre. Illness, disorganisation, must be remedied in the immaterial centre and replaced by newly-established organisation. Medicines in immaterial dilution act on the immaterial centre.

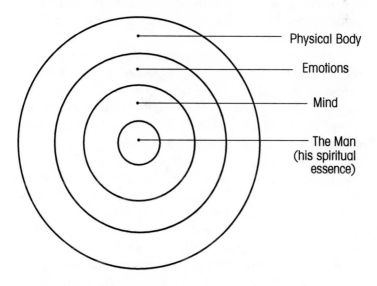

It is important in this respect to realise that the centre is not a perfect soul, even if it is located in the heavenly (spiritual)

level of being. Individually, it may even be quite imperfect and its imperfection should be treated, because it is responsible for illness in our level of perception—in our mind and physical body. We should recall that, according to Swedenborg, there are several higher (heavenly) levels and that these are organised hierarchically according to their level of perfection. They are not entirely separate from each other, but one derives from another. The level of perfection declines downwards.

Hering had already established the rule, obtained from observing people's reactions to homeopathic medicine in non-material potency, that the first area to be cured after an accurately prescribed, holistically-acting medicine, is the mind, which is closest to the immaterial centre. After that come the emotions and only then does the therapeutic wave reach the physical organs. These also are cured on a hierarchical basis, beginning with the central organs that are vital for life, such as the heart, and which are closest in the hierarchy to the individual spiritual centre (which, however, is mutable and certainly not perfect).

In the nineteenth century, America was a deeply spiritual country and the majority of its population shared a profound religiosity. Perhaps this was influenced by the tradition of the Pilgrim Fathers on the Mayflower, and through the founders of the United States, Washington, Jefferson and Franklin, who were Rosicrucians and Freemasons (it is interesting to note that Hahnemann was also a Mason). Swedenborg's teaching also found a warmer welcome in the USA than anywhere else. Indeed, at the end of the nineteenth century homeopaths, heavily influenced by Swedenborg, were in many places more numerous than those doctors who practised normal, materialistic medicine. It was therefore entirely natural that the majority of American homeopaths should believe, in accordance with paragraph nine of Hahnemann's *Organon*, that a precisely prescribed remedy in highly non-material potency has a positive effect not only on the state of the physical organs but firstly on the fine-matter part, the spiritual part of man, and thereby ultimately also on his next birth (passage of consciousness) to the heavenly realms etc. Although this was not mentioned in homeopathic medical books this was a certainty, logically stemming from homeopathic philosophy. Homeopathy and the use of highly diluted substances, the "*spiritual*" forces latent in the medicines (Hahnemann), is thus in essence a spiritual belief system. The holistic effect of the immaterial medicine—focused primarily on the immaterial, hierarchically organised defining sphere of man—does not only include raising the material body to a higher level of health. Its primary function is to raise consciousness (the spirit, soul, mind—whichever term you are easiest with) to a higher spiritual level, from which the dependent physical forms improve as a matter of course.

Highly potentised—diluted—substances act on the non-material centre, the internal Man, according to the resonance principle. When you place two identically tuned tuning forks side by side, and tap one, the other also hums. When you place two differently tuned tuning forks next to each other and tap one the other doesn't even vibrate. In the first instance there is resonance, in the second, not. We search for a medicine that has the closest possible degree of resonance to that of the patient. This then is able in non-material potency to make the patient's non-material part reverberate in his own original (healthy) melody. This is only possible if the medicine is similarly (or identically) tuned. (There even used to be a homeopathic journal called *Resonance*.) The term resonance leads directly to the term frequency. The tuning forks must be tuned to an identical frequency, the number of vibrations per second. Even the slightest variance in the frequency will mean that repeated, firm taps will cause only a slight resonance in the second tuning fork. This, however, rings in its original frequency, and not in the frequency of the other tuning fork. If the frequencies are not similar there will be no resonance.

We thus have a man with his individual frequency, the frequency of his personal string stretched between heaven and earth (or rather between several degrees of heaven and earth) and we are looking for a similar frequency in nature that will resonate with him, that will be similar to him. We recognise a substance with this frequency by the fact that it causes certain symptoms, temporary changes in the mental and physical body in healthy people who take part in homeopathic provings (trials in which substances are tested on human beings). These were recorded in a series of texts collectively known as the "Homeopathic Materia Medica". By comparing our patients' cases with the Materia Medica, we homeopaths find that each patient's symptoms (or the symptoms produced by his non-material organisational system—(the *dynamis*)) accord with a specific medicine and no other. This means that the medicine must have similar frequency characteristics as the spiritual *dynamis* of the patient, producing similar symptoms. Through resonance, the medicine is then able, when diluted to fine-matter level, to elevate the patient's inner fine-matter vibrational centre, the *dynamis*, to a higher (original) vibration level, and allow the entire, slowly collapsing and fading system to return to its original harmony. The illness, the disease, never has a local origin, but invariably signals an error, a shortcoming in the non-material organisational centre. The illness, although perceived as negligible or local, is always a problem of the centre and therefore of the whole.

A homeopathic Repertory exists that gives an alphabetically organised list of symptoms, illnesses, problems and human characteristics and for each such category/symptom (of which there are tens of thousands) provides a list of remedies that include such a symptom in its picture. This helps us find the appropriate, most similar remedy for the whole person from among the hundreds described in the Materia Medica. This has the chance to resonate in homeopathic dilution with the higher, fine-matter states of our "string"—the patient. In addition to the image of the string suggested by the Rosicrucians and the Sufis, I would propose the image of a pendulum, fixed somewhere above in the most ethereal spheres and freely vibrating downwards, with the subtlest impulse upwards causing a great change in the pendulum's downward swing in the gross-matter sphere. Or we may employ a comparison with an electron ray in a television picture: the tiniest variation at its source causes a significant change in the picture on the screen. The cause of everything that happens in the system (organism) rests primarily in the fine-matter sphere, from which everything radiates downwards.

4. More about Vibrations

Vibrations are everything. This is the message of modern quantum physics as well as wave theory, and in the era of television it is an idea that is comprehensible to everyone. Even the most romantic or most violent, the most intelligent and the most stupid television programmes, the most popular television beauties and most sympathetic politicians are only vibrations in the television itself, waves, electric oscillations, the effect of an electron ray on the television screen. And in reality? Again, vibrations of light perceived by the eye, vibrations of sound perceived by the ear, vibrations of pressure perceived by touch... Contemporary science has arrived at the same conclusion as Taoism—that all reality is composed of vibrations, oscillations. But oscillations of what exactly? The question sometimes arouses contradictory responses. Oscillations of subatomic particles, the ether, time-space, yin and yang? Ultimately, perhaps, they can be reduced to the vibrations of consciousness, or more exactly the mind, as Buddhists have maintained for thousands of years. In the teaching of Abhidhamma Buddhists say that all reality is composed of separate segments, of "thought-moments" that are distinguished through the magnifying glass of concentrated meditation. There may be several billion such moments in a single second and between them a small gap—nothing. It recalls a window on a strip of film. A sort of quantum of the mind. Reality is made up of frequencies of the mind.

Is this subjectivism? Or the opposite? That the world isn't created by the mind, but is an entity independent of us? The idea of an objective world, specific to so-called Cartesian science, originated from a purely religious premise posited in the seventeenth century by René Descartes, and by others before him, that the world had been created by an objective God and therefore must be entirely objective and independent of the observer. This proceeds from the wholly unfounded idea that the observer, called the "scientist", is not an active part of the observed world, and may therefore evaluate it from a detached position. In reality, if we think about it seriously, no-one has yet proven that something exists beyond the mind. Just as it has yet to be proven that any such thing as "objective mind" exists.

Even contemporary physicists now believe that the observing subject is part of the process observed, and not a sort of "objective observer". For example, in the theory of "superstrings". This theory also claims that material particles are similar to oscillating mini-strings. Isn't this an interesting terminological conjunction with Rosicrucians and Sufis? And so everything returns to the old truth of the Buddhists, Taoists and others, that everything is in the mind. And in consciousness, which is obviously part of the mind. The mind clearly also has unconscious aspects (see Freud, Jung etc.) of which we only become aware when they surface in consciousness. The only real and direct and incontrovertible truth about so-called reality is that what isn't in consciousness cannot even be mentioned. As soon as we say that "something" does not exist this "something" already exists in consciousness or at least the unconscious. It's a mistake to say that something is "only" in the mind, "only" in consciousness; the mind is enormous and without limits. Its component parts are the so-called "natural laws" of contemporary science. It contains all potential possibilities and may fix on something according to the "governing love" (Swedenborg) or "craving" (Buddha).

According to Buddhists the world is created by the mind and is composed of moments of thought. Or of vibrations or frequencies of consciousness. They said this two and a half thousand years before our scientists reached the same conclusions. These latter narrowed it down just to matter, one of the phenomena of the mind[1], and began to call it quantum physics.

From the accounts of highly-developed individuals it also appears that the higher a person's consciousness reaches, the higher he focuses his attention, the finer are the vibrations and the smaller the difference between the individual and the general. In the highest spheres there exists an area of common thought and consciousness. This is where the vibrations reach their highest frequency. The feeling of individuality and separation from others increases downwards to the lower, gross-matter states, characterised by a fall in frequency. The higher one's attention is focused the more the individual consciousness is able to fuse with the consciousness of "others", with the universe, and the lesser one's individuality. Ultimately, strong feelings of individuality, separation and egoism, combined with great suffering, struggle, increased uncertainty etc., are qualities of these lower states.

Illness and suffering originate and flourish when our spiritual organising principle, our attention, consciousness—and with it also our organism, which is wholly dependent thereon—fall into the lower frequency states. The human body, created by high-frequency patterns in the fine-matter sphere, losing the support and sustenance of these high frequencies, is torn away from them and falls into the lower states, into entropy, and the coordination of functions and organs is lost. Cells, for example, can multiply without coordination, a state we refer to as cancer. The immune system begins to fight itself without coordination leading to auto-immune disorders such as eczema, asthma etc. At a mental level, this process is accompanied by anxiety, or the consciousness that the mind and the body are losing their sustenance from above, and becoming distanced from their ideal, the frequency pattern that exists above. And that, losing contact with it, they begin to decline.

---

[1]   Our feelings and perception—*see* Panca-khandhá, "The Five Groups of Clinging" of the Buddhist Pali canon.

From an ethical viewpoint, this process leads downwards to egoism, a focus on one's own problems, blaming others, an unpleasant or even horrific feeling of alienation from others—but chiefly from the higher frequency sphere, where we are all much closer to each other.

From the point of view of man and his health, much may depend on which frequencies he focuses his attention on.

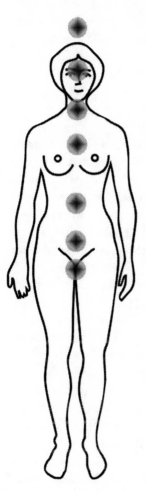

Where attention is focused on effective love (Swedenborg and Buddha), compassion, or on God, who symbolises these qualities for us, the overall frequency of the organism (the secondary, derived frequencies of body and mind) may increase. This is the source of "mysterious" healing through meditation, auto-suggestion etc.

The frequency of consciousness and the organism may also be increased by a potentised, highly-diluted substance which is close in frequency to the relevant organism and is therefore capable at a fine-matter level of resonating with it and reactivating the original or healthy frequency.

In the body the frequency hierarchy corresponds to the system of chakras, which are kinds of energy vortexes in the body described by ancient Indian philosophy. These seven energy centres are related to various vibrational levels in life. The lowest chakra symbolises the relationship to matter, to the earth, to the lowest frequencies; in respect to people the symbolism is of money. The second lowest chakra is the sexual sphere. The chakra of the solar plexus has a strong relation to social success. The heart chakra expresses love; the throat chakra communication; the chakra between the eyebrows relates to higher states of mind and the chakra located above the crown of the head connects us to the highest spiritual states, from where the higher organisational frequencies from the fine-matter sphere flow to us. Some chakras can be closed, while others are active and people concentrate their attention on them and behave at a mental and physical level accordingly.

In recent times, people have focused their attention pre-dominantly on the lower energy levels, strongly supported for example by the media, advertising or the programmes of polit-ical parties. All these social manifestations act almost exclu-sively at the level of the lowest chakras; they reduce people's attention to the lowest frequency levels of existence—mate-rial goods, money, chemically-modified foodstuffs, egoism and violence. This further reduces the overall frequency of the organism, which easily declines into illness. Nowadays, peo-ple suffer from far more chronic or incurable illnesses than at any time previously. They are increasingly alienated from the higher frequency sphere from which they originate. Yang, however, inevitably induces a Yin reaction and so today more people than ever before are again seeking that relation with the high frequency sphere. That is why, despite the powerful forces of destruction acting in the lower frequencies and drag-ging man down, there is such interest in homeopathy, Bud-dhism, alternative healing and spirituality; in re-establishing a personal relationship with the higher creative sphere. The terms "new religiosity" or "New Age" are sometimes given to this unorganised movement, which nevertheless comprises very significant numbers of people in the West.

A certain frequency can create entirely specific mate-rial structures or forms. This is testified to by experiments in physics conducted by the Swiss philosopher Hans Jenny. He sprinkled fine sand on a sheet of metal and dispersed it uniformly. Then he oscillated the sheet. Certain frequencies caused specific arrangements in pictures. When the frequency was changed another picture appeared which corresponded to the altered frequency. The experiment makes it abundantly clear that a certain frequency can create corresponding shapes and forms in a particular environment (in this experiment using sand). As an analogy, we may easily imagine that the human body with all its organs is also created and maintained by certain creative, organising frequencies.

The highest hierarchical frequencies have the greatest creative influence and exist in a super-sensory sphere. Our external, physical senses are turned to the material world and are able to perceive on its gross-matter, low frequency, to which they are tuned. They can't perceive (with the exception of the mind itself, which the Buddhists refer to as the sixth sense) fine-matter, hierarchically higher frequencies. The same applies to scientific instruments.

As has already been said, in our world the gradual descent to lower frequencies, to greater alienation, individuality and egoism, seems to be natural, widespread and unavoidable. For some people this process unfolds slowly, imperceptibly; for others it is rapid. Let us recall the Biblical story of the expulsion of Adam and Eve from Paradise. This symbolises the descent from the fine-matter, ethically higher and blissful sphere of higher union, where there is nothing to hide, to the gross-matter world of contradictions, personal hardship and alienation (isolation).

Illness is disorganisation originating in the lower levels of the superior creative sphere. The opposite way is possible, but only ever on the basis of concentrated effort and the overcoming of downward tendencies.

As a person ages his central frequency falls relative to the intensity with which he is exposed to the lower, gross-matter environment, the sphere of low thought frequencies, fear, hatred, envy, disgust etc. The impact of the original, internal creative frequency on the associated lower frequencies that envelop it weakens; ultimately they may lose almost all contact with each other, which entails growing disharmony, disorganisation (e.g. cancer), decline and the death of these lower, derived frequencies, whose energy still has to be channelled from those above. The deteriorating lower physical frequencies have already fallen too far, have become too distant from the central frequency and can no longer resonate accordingly, thereby losing the vibrational energy source. As a result it terminates and dies. But it is precisely the lower frequencies perceived by the senses that are commonly understood as the person, or individual. In fact, however, this refers only to the "external" or "natural" man, as Swedenborg says. Man's higher and more internal central frequency continues to exist, with attention/consciousness being focused on it once again in the moment of death, when the gross-matter frequency—the organs—succumb to the effects of entropy. In time, these central, high frequencies create a new body by interacting with the frequencies of the new environment. Here, environment should be understood to mean also its parents or generative cells. If the central frequency really is extremely high (it was not depleted during the course of life or, indeed, it was amplified through the high-frequency stimulus of love, wisdom or a precise, highly-potentised medicine) the new body is created at a higher frequency in a higher (heavenly) world with a lower level of suffering, a weaker illusion of individuality, greater love and connection with others, and tolerance. If, on the other hand, the person's central frequency was strongly affected and therefore significantly reduced by the lower frequencies of hatred, the desire to harm others and similar motivations, the new body may come into being in the lower world full of low vibrations and generating higher levels of suffering and uncertainty than in its previous existence.

In this way, the entire world of interactions, perceived as ethical, religious, objective or subjective, may also appear merely as an impersonal world of vibrations. Buddha once revealed that in their essence these are the impersonal vibrations of the mind. Matter, substance, is also the product of the linking of the sphere of the senses with the mind; it is part of the sphere of the mind which includes everything and is the cause of everything. The ancient principle, known to all idealistic philosophical systems—the primacy of mind over matter. Matter is a vibration and is also the product of the mind. Through separation from the world of vibrations, and also therefore the mind, the world retreats, and with it, suffering. For us, this is an unimaginable state of nirvana, a state neither of existence or non-existence, a state of knowing everything. In Buddhist philosophy it is a state of absolute health.

The causal ties between phenomena, people, events and so on, are not horizontal, as understood by contemporary science and common sense, which focus only on low frequencies of matter, but rather vertical and hierarchical. Phenomena and people meet in an elevated, spiritual, fine-matter sphere of higher vibrations. If Hahnemann says that the cause of health and illness is in the higher, spiritual sphere he means exactly this. Infection is not spread by bacilli or viruses etc., but by dissonances and disharmony in the higher sphere. A bacillus is a creature, happily living off the products of diseased dissonance (toxins, waste matter) and tissues weakened by dissonance. A highly-diluted medicine resonating with the immaterial creative frequency restores order and harmony and the "disease-making" micro-organisms depart, deprived of the means necessary for their existence. Any chronic illness, from hay fever to serious heart disease or madness, means that the organism is to some degree severed from the influence of the high-frequency, fine-matter (in materialistic terminology immaterial) organisational vibrational principle of the Inner

Man (Swedenborg, Kent), sustaining or actually moment by moment creating the individual material body.

Summary:
- The universe is built on the relations of relevant frequencies and resonances.
- Very high (far higher than the highest frequency detectable by a material instrument) spiritual or fine-matter frequencies are the authors of both lower thought frequencies and even lower material frequencies.
- Very high spiritual frequencies thus have a creative character.
- The organism is constantly being formed from and sustained by the fine, high-frequency creative sphere.
- The organism's frequency falls due to interaction with the environment, in particular as a result of stress, whether psychological, social, ecological or otherwise, or simply through the passing of time, with resulting illness. The frequency can be increased through resonance with a substance tuned on a similar frequency, if this has been elevated to the high-frequency, fine-matter creative sphere through being potentised (homeopathically diluted). A deterioration in health (even local) always involves the person's fine-matter sphere and is generated from there as its malfunction.
- A therapeutic substance is by dilution with water elevated to the higher frequency fine-matter sphere; the more it is diluted, the higher the frequency sphere it reaches.
- The homeopath's overriding objective is to find a substance that resonates with the relevant individual's creative frequency, and then to provide this substance in homeopathically diluted form. In so doing, the entire organism attains a higher frequency and a higher state of organisation, of health. It then resonates better with

the higher creative frequencies that bear an ideal model or structure of the man (Swedenborg and Kent write 'Man').

- The more a person's frequency drops below the highest creative frequencies, the greater the suffering and chronic tendency to illness.
- The more a person's frequency drops below the highest creative frequencies, the less capable the organism is of maintaining its original structure. With the fall in the central frequency this begins to disintegrate, to change into another, less organised structure corresponding to its lower frequency.
- Each frequency creates an entirely specific structure in each specific environment. It is therefore possible for the fall in frequency to cause not only illness, mistakes or confusion in the original structure of thought and organs, but also (after death) rebirth in a lower frequency state that corresponds, for example, to the animal structure of body and mind. Lower frequency states result in states of increased suffering, uncertainty and turbulence.
- Existence in higher frequency states than those that are manifest in our world is called "heavenly". There are frequency levels referred to in the terminology of various religions as "heaven". According to Buddhists, Swedenborg, yoga, the Kabbalah, Islam and other systems, there are many of these, organised hierarchically "one above the other". One derives from another, the lower from the higher. We could add: some are higher and some lower according to the frequency height of their states.
- Upon the death of the individual, the low, material frequency of the body separates from the person's consciousness located in the highest frequency levels. The material frequency terminates and the material structure starts to disintegrate. This is an equivalent state to

those described in near-death experiences that occur in states of clinical death or the first phase of dying. Where it proved possible to resuscitate the dying persons they have spoken of their experiences, in which they were able to observe their dead, separating body from afar, their consciousness no longer tied to the body. In these states they experienced a sense of lightness and relief and went through a sort of very rapid film of their life, replayed backwards, i.e. they went through the frequency states of the mind which they had experienced since birth. Issue No. 359 of the respected medical journal *The Lancet*, published in December 2001, contained a statistical study by the Dutch doctor Pim van Lomel, which claimed that "45% of adults and more than 85% of children who had undergone life-threatening illnesses had experienced near-death experiences". He explains that most of those adults who could not claim near-death experiences had forgotten about it. So, even by the criteria of contemporary medical science, a high percentage of people passing through the first stage of death underwent and described experiences linked to the separation of the higher thought frequencies from the material body. The aforementioned study confirms (even if it doesn't explicitly state) that man is a multi-dimensional being, existing contemporaneously in different, hierarchically connected (frequency) levels. Among other things, the article stated: "Nothing suggests that these experiences, which followed the stoppage of the heart, were caused by psychological, neurophysiological or physiological factors."

When considering these matters we should always bear in mind that all people who have reached high levels of spiritual insight spoke the languages of their time only so as to be understood by others. Human speech is a symbolic instrument that derives from expressions which are valid for normal daily experience. When a physicist speaks of a "field", he doesn't mean a field of potatoes or wheat but something else. When we speak about a vibration we imagine an ordinary, metal oscillating tuning fork, or a sort of sinusoidal curve. But people's life experience changes and terminology and technology become outdated. It is therefore quite possible also to say: vibrations or frequencies are probably the best model (or perhaps metaphor?) by which contemporary man may understand the aforementioned effects of diluted substances on man's higher sphere and consequently on his lower spheres. Nevertheless, it is possible to use the medicines in accordance with the outlined principles and rules of treatment without trying to understand anything—it is not essential. We shall thereby avoid terminological and ideological, if not directly religious, disputes. Buddha provides an excellent parable: On a battlefield a man is struck by a poisoned arrow. A physician is called to remove the arrow. The injured man, however, asks that before they remove the arrow they tell him who shot it, at what distance, who were the man's brothers and sisters... Before they can tell him everything he wants to know the poison enters his body and he dies. Instead of theorising it is better to remove the arrow as quickly as possible. Some of us, however, love theory and can't live without it.

5. Finding an Equivalent Vibration Pattern

Every person, as well as every creature and object, has its own vibration pattern, a superior creative frequency. This is Swedenborg's "Inner Man" and Hahnemann's "dynamis" or "vital force". The Buddhist conviction that the world is created by the mind (frequencies of the mind) corresponds in Swedenborg's system to the opinion that the world and universe is Man, or his mind, as Swedenborg's system concerns only the mind. Angels (in Buddhism devas) and beings from the higher worlds in general are also finer and ethically higher likenesses of Man, or of his more abstract states of mind. When Swedenborg talks about them he works with the theory of frequency, of waves. In his book *Heaven and Hell* he writes that because he was on the same wavelength he perceived their (i.e. angels in heaven) conversations as he would any other normal conversation.

The basic vibration structure or pattern is the same at both the finest and highest frequency level and at the lowest. It is a few octaves higher in the fine-matter state (soul, spirit, higher states of mind, the organisational immaterial principle in man etc.). It drops some octaves for derived states of mind, for psychological states, and drops again for physical organs, the human body with its basic building elements, cells, genes and molecules. But the melody remains the same. In this respect we should recall the central proposition of alchemy ascribed to Hermes Trismegistus: "As above, so below". This means that all the forms and functions of the physical body and lower and higher levels of mind have their model in a higher, fine-matter (Swedenborg would say *heavenly*) frequency state. This applies not only to properly functioning organs but also to those that function badly, wrongly, which are out of harmony and are sick. Before disharmony manifests itself at a bodily level as chronic eczema, it has to appear in the fine-matter sphere and from there it radiates to the physical organ. If, in order to treat a skin complaint, we prescribe a medicine that only works at a superficial level the problem will remain unsolved as it is constantly renewed from the high frequency sphere from which it derives and where the complaint has its source, and from where the part of the body affected is created. Homeopaths have always said that they cure the internal cause of the illness. At this point I would like to include some direct quotations from Hahnemann's *Organon* (English edition, Cooper Publishing, Blaine, Washington 1982). These brilliantly and precisely describe the situation I have outlined above. In addition to paragraph nine, which I have already quoted, I should add the following:

§10 "Without the vital force the material organism is unable to feel, or act, or maintain itself. Only because of the immaterial being (vital principle, vital force) that animates it in health and in disease can it feel and maintain its vital functions."

§12 "It is only the pathologically untuned vital force that causes diseases. The pathological manifestations accessible to our senses express all the internal changes, i.e., the whole pathological disturbance of the *dynamis*: they reveal the whole disease. Conversely, the cessation through treatment of all the symptoms, i.e., the disappearance of all perceptible deviations from health, necessarily implies that the vital principle has recovered its integrity and therefore that the whole organism has returned to health."

For the sake of clear understanding in the relevant context (not in any way to change the meaning or from a desire to improve on the classics), all you have to do is replace the term "vital force" with the term "higher creative frequency" or "Inner Man", and the core of Hahnemann's teaching combines very logically with the Buddhist vision of things (highfrequency vibrations of the mind) as well as with Swedenborg's outlook (both preceded Hahnemann's formulations).

Whereas paragraphs 9 and 10 teach us about the basic hierarchical system that causes man and his organism to function in sickness and in health, paragraph 12 directly refers to the method of distinguishing, of diagnosing the "internal" illness, and therefore also of determining the medicine. Disharmony in the higher, non-material sphere produces disharmony in the lower, bodily sphere, which is "evident to our senses", sensually discernible. If we assemble *all* the available data about the sick person (*Organon*, paragraph 18) from this sensually discernible sphere, all his personality, his mental and emotional characteristics and an overall description of physical dissonance, of the disease, of all his ailments and diseases, we shall learn how the non-material creative frequency, the productive state, looks. Melody and disharmony are the same "as above, so below".

After the type of disharmony has been discerned, diagnosed, the treatment phase can begin—i.e. finding the right medicine. In order for it to be therapeutic this must be similar to the specific disharmony: it must be able to produce a similar disharmony in the healthy person. This is the fundamental rule of homeopathy, the famous *"similia similibus curantur"*, "like cures like". But how do we find the right medicine? First, we conduct provings using a variety of potentised substances on healthy people. Any changes (sometimes very subtle changes) that the potentised substances (plants, minerals, animal tissue or fluids etc.) induce in the healthy volunteers—provers—are carefully recorded and published.

For example, the Lachesis snake poison may cause clogging of the veins in the lower limbs and inflammation of the throat, which moves from the left to the right side of the throat and is soothed by cool drinks. The prover may experience choking sensations, but also groundless feelings of jealousy, garrulousness and lack of concentration. While using the substance in its raw state may even result in death, the application of a potentised substance causes a moderate reaction that quickly passes, "strengthening the health of the prover" (Hahnemann). Patients who suffer repeatedly from inflammation of the throat of the aforementioned type, who also experience feelings of jealousy and are unusually talkative, can therefore be treated with potentised, highly-diluted Lachesis. The substance, however, is not restricted to throat inflammations; it also reduces jealousy and strengthens the organism's resistance to external stress, whether psychological or physical (infection, pollution etc.). The treatment never concerns a single ailment; it always and fundamentally applies to an overall change, produced by a positive change in the person's centrally-acting creative frequency. We can say that the frequency and vibrational pattern for the patient and the Lachesis medicine are similar: *Similia similibus curantur*. If the patient and the medicine are similar, there will be resonance at the high fine-matter level; the organism's high frequency level will again reverberate in its original tone and cause the lower level, linking mental and physical, to return to normal, bringing about a gradual improvement in health. The greater the similarity between patient and medicine, the more intense and complete is the resonance and the therapeutic reaction. In other words, the greater the similarity of the patient and his feeling with the feelings recorded by the tested persons during the proving of the medicine. The medicine's vibrational pattern described in the Materia Medica is therefore not a list of the substance's qualities *per se*, for example sulphur or Lachesis; instead it expresses exclusively the relation of the human organism and human psyche to this substance. This means the resonance relation obtained during the medicine's proving.

From schoolboy experiments with tuning forks we are well aware of how, the greater the difference between the reverberating fork and the resonating fork, the harder and more frequent the strokes have to be in order to achieve resonance. Homeopathy works according to the same principle. If we gather information about the client on a random basis, and exclusively from the physical sphere, and neglect for example his salient mental characteristics, we will acquire an inaccurate picture of the creative frequency and choose a medicine that is only partially similar and which does not resonate sufficiently. We are then forced to provide repeated doses of the medicine, or to change it frequently and combine it with others in order to achieve any sort of therapeutic reaction, at least at a local level. If the medicine is tuned completely differently to its recipient nothing will happen, there will be no response and things will continue upon their original course. It is well known that during a homeopathic proving only some provers will react (those who have the nearest tuning) while others will undergo practically no change whatsoever. When, however, we are able to obtain the important characteristics from the mental sphere, which is the closest to the person's creative central frequency, we shouldn't pay too much attention to the peripheral and physical symptoms that need to be treated. The medicine, chosen exactly according to the symptoms of the mind (see Rajan Sankaran: *The Spirit of Homeopathy, The Soul of Remedies*) will resonate with the centre and will cure the whole, including the physical problems. A single application will act for several months. It will also gradually improve or cure chronic, long-term and deep-seated ailments. A frequency of medicine selected in this way will also cure acute illnesses.

Like a chronic ailment, an acute illness is primarily caused by disharmony or a reduction in frequency in the person's fundamental creative fine-matter sphere, from which all of the organism's manifestations, psychological or physical, healthy or diseased, derive. If somebody who has a temporary disposition to contract influenza meets a person who has influenza he will begin to resonate with that person and will also catch the flu. Another person doesn't have an internal disposition to flu and won't catch it from a sick person, even though he has inhaled the viruses as well. As soon as the internal disposition of the sick person is remedied using a homeopathic treatment that resonates with the centre, the acute illness swiftly disappears and bacteria and viruses no longer find fertile ground in which to multiply and form which to feed off.

When we think about it, we find that our whole life is based on resonance. We don't only infect people with illness but also with happiness and positive moods, if this is inside us and others are tuned to perceive it. If we like someone it means that our personality resonates with him or her, that it reverberates within us, that in it we find a part of ourselves. That it is on our frequency. A beautiful picture resonates in us through the frequencies of its colours and forms; beautiful music elevates us through the frequencies of its tones; a work of philosophy is on the same frequency of reflection as our mind. It applies to relations between people, to art and politics, social activities. There are also many things that we either don't perceive at all or which we reject. Here there is no resonance, or if so it is negligible—it is not our frequency, it is not tuned to us, it passes us by.

The term "frequency" should not be confused with the term "energy". The first signifies quality and the second quantity. The first creates shapes, feelings, forms etc.—it is creative—whereas the second is linked to volume and strength and is derivative. Volume and strength are secondary. We can smash the tuning fork with a hammer and still we can't get the second fork to reverberate if it isn't on the same or similar frequency. The attempt to replace resonance with energy when treating patients commonly increases the suffering and creates greater entropy, particularly with regard to treatment, but also in politics and other matters.

6. Seeking Resonance

A specific, characteristic vibration pattern or structure creates (firstly at a fine-matter, and then a secondary, material level) a specific, typical personality structure, an organism with all its organs, specific behaviour and specific suffering—pathology. Illness is not something inorganic, external, accidental, it is an inherent part of the system, the logical consequence of a development towards ever greater disorganisation, disharmony and entropy. If we prescribe a resonating medicine in a fine-matter, highly diluted potency, the error will be remedied in the high fine-matter sphere, which can only be reached by the potentised substance. This, because it is tuned similarly to the individual concerned, causes the fine-matter sphere to sound again in its original melody or frequency structure. Let's recall the similar tuning forks. If we strike one, the second also rings, but in its own original frequency, not that of its partner, which is the source of the resonance. The renewed or rather strengthened or refreshed creative fine-matter frequency causes the organism's original, healthy structure belonging to the original frequency to renew itself. The illness, the disorganisation that manifests itself at the material level discernible to the senses, then subsides as it is replaced by the organism's healthy, original structure, whose source is in the fine-matter sphere. This is an active process. The essential thing is to find the appropriate, resonating medicine. The more this is attuned to the relevant individual, the more it can evoke the resonance and thereby cure the individual concerned.

Samuel Hahnemann started searching[2] for a resonating or similar medicine at the end of the eighteenth century with his

---

[2]   For the purposes of this book, whose main subject matter is autopathy, I describe only the bases of homeopathic philosophy and methodology. More detailed information can be found in my book *Homeopathy, More Than A Cure*, Alternativa, Prague.

proving of *China officinalis*, or the bark of the cinchona tree. The choice of this first substance, a plant, for a homeopathic proving has its roots in the medical practice of the period, which used this substance in a raw state to cure malaria. Hahnemann realised that the substance caused the same symptoms in a healthy person as those recorded by people suffering from malaria. He deduced that it was precisely because the medicine was similar to malaria and produced a state similar to malaria that it was able to cure the disease. He thus discovered the principle of similarity.

Hahnemann later realised that acute pathological problems are not accidental but derive instead from a general, deep-seated pathological disposition that is common to everybody and which is innate. He called this disposition "miasm", which means contamination. A person who has a low pathological disposition has a negligible disposition to illness and will not fall ill even in the middle of the severest epidemic. From his enormous medical experience, Hahnemann thus concluded that the basic objective of treatment should be to remedy this general disposition to illness, the miasm. If it were possible to find a medicine that corresponded to all sides of the personality, the patient's entire vibrational pattern, a cure could be provided for all illnesses that stemmed from it. An effective cure would render the person healthy and resistant to negative influences. Chronic and long-term illnesses would disappear. Hahnemann distinguished between three basic types of miasm, namely sycotic, (for which the main medicines are *Thuja* and *Medorrhinum*), psoric, (*Sulphur* and *Psorinum*), and syphilitic (*Mercurius* and *Syphilinum*). We see that in relation to the main theme of this book, autopathy, every miasm is connected to a medicine taken from the human body. Hahnemann's miasms have certain basic qualities defined by the general character of the ailment. The sycotic miasm is characterised by over-production, surplus (e.g. warts, cysts, obesity); the psoric miasm's distinguishing feature is an insufficiency of something, decline and disappearance, while the syphilitic miasm is characterised by destruction and disintegration.

Subsequent authors added a list of other types of miasms and significantly complicated the whole process by declaring that a single person may have all the miasms at once. Miasms therefore have no special value in determining a specific remedy but do have an important philosophical influence. Hahnemann says that this is a fundamental pathological disposition that has to be cured, instead of treating its specific manifestations. This is a lofty ideal and certainly based on true and empirically verifiable facts. The theory was developed over time, most importantly in Kent's work where he talks about the constitution. Kent divides medicines into two basic categories: "deep-acting" and "superficially-acting" medicines. Deep-acting medicines are able to resonate with the internal organisational system, with the inner Man, while the second category is distant from Man's organising centre and through its resonance affects only some localised peripheral parts, organs, specific ailments etc. The first category is able to affect the entire constitution, the fundamental make-up of a person, and thereby to cure all pathological elements contained in the relevant constitution. The second category does not have this capability, although it may have a temporary impact on the miasm's local manifestations.

According to Kent, a medicine that can cure the constitution, or the entire miasm that is producing the health problems—the illness—is a "constitutional medicine". The highest goal of Kent's homeopathy is to cure the constitution, the whole, the Inner Man, or to uproot the miasm, as Hahnemann sought to do. In other words, to establish a permanent state of inner health and the external health that results from it. The beginning of the *Organon* proclaims the same ideal, for example in paragraph 2: "The highest ideal of therapy is to restore health rapidly, gently, permanently." Both writers, Hahnemann and Kent, then proceed to state categorically that a miasm is not (despite meaning "contamination") a passive and quantitative element but rather a qualitative "dynamis" or "Inner Man" that succumbs to disorganisation, entropy and confusion. Miasms are understood to be disharmony as opposed to the harmony that is health.

So, a homeopath's work consists primarily of seeking the constitutional medicine that most closely resonates with the centre, with a person's central frequency. He finds it by examining not only the pathology but all its circumstances, including past ailments and psychology and social behaviour, and then comparing this with the description in the Materia Medica. As a result, illnesses of all sorts acquired over the person's lifetime gradually disappear, and the healed centre sets about the long process of re-establishing order in the hierarchically lower levels.

In order to make it absolutely clear what this means, I shall describe a case from my own homeopathic practice:

On 1 June 2000, I was visited by a forty-one year old man of robust build but with a brow furrowed by worry. His main problems were concentrated in his lungs, bronchial tubes and tonsils. He often had a stabbing pain in his chest; this had been at its most serious the previous winter when it had been so severe that he had had to lie down, unable to move, and hadn't even been able to eat. Every winter it got worse. He suffered from a persistent, chronic cough, which was aggravated during cool weather and outside in cold air, when he also had problems breathing. If he drank something cold his tonsils immediately hurt and quantities of phlegm were produced, causing him to cough. He had first experienced problems in his throat and bronchial tubes twenty years previously, after recovering from a sore throat. He also suffered from a painful knee, particularly when there was a draught in the car, and had done for several years. All these complaints had been unsuccessfully treated by conventional medicine.

In order to gain a fuller picture I asked if he had suffered from any other ailments in the past. This is important when deciding on the type of medicine to treat current health problems, as the same non-material centre (fine-matter vibration pattern) that produced the current pathology is also responsible for other problems of the same type in the past. The more one knows, the better one is able to prescribe a resonating medicine. He told me that as a child and young man he had been extremely healthy and hadn't suffered any illnesses. Some years ago, however, he had suffered back pain, which had extended to his legs. This had got better but had been replaced by repeated headaches.

The information obtained thus far would not be sufficient for a precise prescription. The physical ailments would satisfy the description for hundreds of medicines. Of greater importance is the (general) character of the ailments—meaning their exacerbation by cold weather and drafts. Through a combination of pathology and its general character—the exacerbation of all ailments by cold weather and particularly drafts—we proceed by elimination to a category of some several dozen medicines that include both features in their description.

I then asked about the times of day or night when the ailments made themselves felt or were particularly bad. He told me that the critical time was between 4 and 8 p.m. This is important, as different homeopathic types and medicines (the type of patient and description of the medicine have to correspond) have different critical times in the twenty-four-hour cycle. According to Murphy's *Homeopathic Medical Repertory*, which is my primary source of reference, there are twelve medicines that have an aggravation during this period, while approximately another ten fall. The process of elimination from the original, roughly two thousand, homeopathic types described thus continues and the selection is now narrowed down to a few medicines that have all the aforementioned characteristics of the patient.

Most pertinent to the character of the central frequency,

however, is the individual's own psyche, which is directly influenced by the frequency. I therefore asked about his feelings, emotions and behaviour and I learned that:

He is an extremely anxious person, but tries to hide this from others. At university he didn't sleep at all the night before his examinations. In arguments he remains cool even though inside he is burning up with rage. He tries to dominate and decide for others in matters where he feels competent, particularly at work, where he holds a managerial position. He likes competition both at work and elsewhere because it stimulates him to perform better. He played team sports, football, basketball and hockey and liked all of them, chiefly because of the element of competition. He has had to give them up for health reasons. He has bad Mondays because during the weekends he loses his work rhythm. He sometimes has problems sleeping, waking at three in the morning and then not being able to get back to sleep, particularly on Sunday night. On Monday he also has a bad headache that lasts throughout the day and which is sometimes so intense that it stops him driving. This restricts him in his work duties as his job requires him to spend several hours a day behind the wheel.

This psychological picture is as if drawn directly from the Materia Medica (which isn't always the case in practice) and a comparison with the description in the Materia Medica shows that it corresponds to the medicine *Lycopodium clavatum*, potentised spores of Club Moss. The pathology and general details (general character of the ailments) also match this medicine. The patient also corresponds to the medicine's basic essence, which is to adapt to ever-changing circumstances and successfully to survive in competition with others. When we realise that Cub Moss is the oldest land plant, dating from the Palaeozoic age, where it was dominant, and that it succeeded in adapting to the fundamental changes in climate and surrounding fauna and flora, and in surviving until the present day, we see that even the existence of a plant is dictated by the same essential motive as a person of the *Lycopodium* type. This is why there is such a strong resonance between the plant and a person of its type, a resonance that has healing power.

I recommended *Lycopodium* 200C. The number 200 means the number of centesimal dilutions. The so-called Avogadro limit is reached on the twelfth dilution, which means that statistically from this point onwards no particle of the original substance can occur in the diluted product. He took a single tablet dissolved on the tongue.

Three and a half months later, on 19 September 2000, he came back for a follow-up and took out the notes in which, at my suggestion, he had recorded any important changes in his state of health. I recommend the taking of notes to everyone, irrespective of whether this involves homeopathic or autopathic treatment. People easily forget unpleasant events, pain or fevers—this is a psychological automatism that helps keep us alive. If you had a fever a fortnight ago you would find it very difficult to remember precisely what happened. If the problems pass in a few days you would know nothing about them. And after three months...! The man looked into his notes and read out: "Improvement in sleep. Head doesn't hurt. At the end of June a sharp pain in my back when moving awkwardly; since then occasional pain under my right rib-cage and sometimes on the left. This disappeared of its own accord after two weeks".

My task now was to find whether the patient had experienced these symptoms previously. If he had, this would be good news, as it would mean that he was beginning to experience the previous frequency (qualitative) states that he had passed through before entering his pathology. He was on the road to recovery. We can picture his life's journey as a sort of stairway.

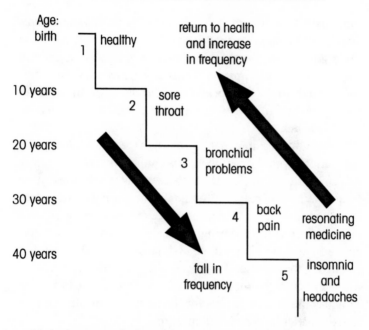

If the organism's frequency state increases following the prescription of the resonating medicine this means that it is passing retroactively through previous physical and psychological symptoms that were linked to the same frequency in the past—in this case back pain. The psyche also returned to a much better, higher state. As a result he now reacts far better to stress, he no longer suffers from headaches and can handle work pressures better. He also says that he feels much better and has a better attitude to life in general.

The nineteenth-century American homeopath Constantine Hering established the rules (today known as the Hering's Laws of Cure) by which the individual progresses following the prescription of the appropriate medicine: *Ailments are cured from within outward*—i.e. there is improvement first in the centrally-located ailments in the most important organs, then in the peripheral organs. In our case, this corresponds to the improvement in the insomnia and headaches during the first phase of treatment. The second law is: *Ailments are cured in the reverse order to that in which they occurred.* A person undergoing homeopathic treatment is gradually relieved of his problems and ailments as his frequency increases. This corresponds to the disappearance of headaches as the final ailment and the temporary return of back pain, which preceded the headaches.

We should also note that the problems recede from the central frequency to the periphery. This only happens in response to a correctly chosen medicine that resonates with the central frequency and increases it. In this way we learn whether a true homeopathic reaction has taken place. If the symptoms do not proceed according to Hering's Laws this means that the medicine was not entirely accurate and has not caused the central frequency to increase. If we discern them at the beginning of treatment after the medicine has been administered this also provides the best prognosis for the treatment of the ailments that the patient has suffered hitherto.

No other medicine was prescribed and the man did not appear again until 3 April 2001, ten months after the medicine had been administered. He said that he hadn't once been ill throughout the entire winter (for the first time in ten years, perhaps even in his life). The chronic cough had disappeared and hadn't once returned, the recurring problems with his throat had passed and all the aforementioned physical ailments had gone too. His Monday blues had disappeared and his sleep had improved; for a long time he hadn't woken in the night as he used to do. He was very satisfied and totally healthy.

He came for another follow-up in September 2001, which merely confirmed the state of health from the previous follow-up.

On 3 January 2002, however, he came to tell me that he had been suffering from headaches for three weeks. Moreover, he had started to wake in the night again and stayed up till dawn.

He felt overstressed at work. What did this mean? After a year and a half the medicine had ceased to have any influence, the resonance of the centre had faded and its frequency had fallen to its previous state at the beginning of treatment. The reduction had been accompanied by a recurrence of the symptoms (in homeopathy we call this a relapse) that corresponded to the falling frequency. This first affected the mind (poor sleep), which is the most closely linked to the central frequency. After that came the centrally-located ailments—headaches—which, located in the central organ, the brain, are hierarchically also closely connected to the centre. Physical ailments—the cough, tonsillitis etc., had not yet followed, but could be expected to appear soon.

In such a situation, it is necessary to renew the resonance with the centre at the highest level. I recommended *Lycopodium* 1M—a thousand-times centesimally diluted preparation. A single tablet was prescribed.

The patient came for a further check up 25 April 2002, at which he told me that four days after taking the tablet he had begun to feel poorly. He had suffered from strong headaches and vomited, he had had to lie down for four days, he felt unsteady when walking and in an X-ray doctors had found a blockage in a cervical vertebra. He woke at three in the night and couldn't get back to sleep. He couldn't concentrate on anything. The highly potentised medicine had resulted in a marked deterioration of the ailments, a process we refer to as a "homeopathic aggravation". A deterioration of existing or previous symptoms that occurs within a few days of administering the medicine means that the organism has reacted and this is understood as a good sign for future development. A deterioration of this sort only occurs after the prescription of a precisely resonating medicine, although this does not always happen. In many cases no aggravation is evident, or if so, it is only very slight and almost indiscernible. (In America, there even used to be an journal called *Homeopathic Aggrava-*

tion). Aggravation only rarely reaches the intensity described. Over the following two weeks everything righted itself. Two months later, the patient was again free of the ailments, including the former chronic complaints; everything was functioning exactly as it should and he felt wonderful. The usual winter coughs and throat ache had not reappeared. He was healthy and very satisfied with the treatment.

The follow-up enabled us to see just how quickly the physical organism responds to the centre's increased fine-matter frequency, passes through its former states and rapidly acquires robust health.

The whole process before and after administering the holistic medicine reminds me somewhat of an inflatable fairground balloon. When we blow it up it is beautifully smooth, healthy. In his youth a person is relatively healthy and without chronic problems; unfortunately this idyll today often ends in babyhood. The invisible interior then starts slowly to depart through leaks caused primarily by its relation with harsh and polluting surroundings and/or rough treatment; the surface of the balloon softens and wrinkles.

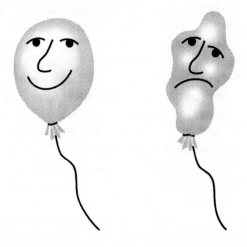

A person becomes accustomed to the wrinkling process and to illness, to faults in this once beautiful, smooth surface. Through the use of traditional medicines, massages and superficially-acting medication he tries to apply cosmetics to the balloon, a sort of plastic surgery, evening out or stretching at least some of the wrinkles. But the air is still decreasing and so when we artificially apply pressure or smooth one side of the balloon the other side suffers all the more. Eventually, we become accustomed to the wrinkles, even if we do not want to. Then someone appears, a homeopath with a constitutional medicine, who instead of evening out the wrinkles blows the balloon up, thereby supplying it with that invisible essence that gives it shape. The surface tautens, the wrinkles disappear, but because the material on the surface around it has hardened, even this process can sometimes be painful, although obviously far more pleasant than the path towards illness. The comparison is simply to remind us that a real cure always applies to the whole, and that beneath the surface there is something invisible that is of essential importance and which provides shape. But because the comparison with a balloon does not exactly correspond to the frequency concept, I would like to refer again to the analogy of the staircase I used earlier. The organism returns to frequency states that it has previously experienced in youth, at a time when it suffered far fewer serious ailments, or even none whatsoever—a time when it was relatively healthy. The organism's external state corresponds to the centre's internal frequency state. Changes in the internal state cause changes in the external state. "As above, so below."

Occasionally, after administering a medicine with a very precise resonance it can happen that a person who has been chronically ill his entire life, afflicted by a variety of complaints, finds hitherto unknown health. This was perhaps what happened in the *Lycopodium* case. The patient is able to reach a higher frequency state than ever before. Spiritually, and then also physically, he comes nearer than ever before to the fine-matter universal frequency known as Man, from which we all, some more perfectly and others less so, derive.

But people are developing constantly, even under influence of a constitutional homeopathic remedy. Let us continue with our *Lycopodium* case:

In August 2004 he told me that his wife, who was attending my seminars of autopathy, gave him seven months ago an *autopathic preparation* in the potency 200C because his problems started to return. Since that time he is without symptoms and moreover he reported that his relations with people improved a lot in the family as well as in his job. It was much easier for him to communicate with people. Further reports I have from his wife: Till April 2006 he took two more autopathic potencies prepared in the Autopathic Bottle. He got 1M in September 2004 because a very slight chronic hay-fever occurring every Spring since his childhood. Than it did not appear for the first time in the course of a hay season. The second dose was in the potency of 2M because of a slight negative mood. His wife reported that he is now (in April 2006) in perfect health and even able to deal better with his inevitable daily problems at work.

The following case is another example of seeking resonance that should bring us a step closer to the main subject of this book, autopathy.

At the end of December 2000, a slim, attractive brunette in her late thirties knocked at my door and told me the following:

Her doctor's official diagnosis was ankylosying spondylitis. She had a stiff back, which gave her a lot of pain, and she suffered from cramp in her muscles. Over the previous three months this had been worse than ever before, even though she had experienced these complaints since the age of eleven. Her knee, wrist and shoulder also hurt her. She was taking anti-rheumatic and other medicines. She was constantly tired, particularly in the evening; later in the evening it improved a little. She suffered badly from flatulence and constipation alternating with diarrhoea. She felt that things were going from bad to worse; recently she had also slept badly, taking a long time to fall asleep and then often waking up and being unable to fall asleep again, even though she needed to sleep so badly due to her tiredness. She was very tearful, breaking into tears at the slightest cause, sometimes several times a day, including at the parents' evening at her child's school. She clutched a handkerchief in her hand as she told me about her problems and the tears ran down her face. Although she had serious physical ailments she felt that the main problem and source of her suffering was psychological. She felt enormous internal tension and her tiredness was also probably psychological in origin; sometimes she was so tired that she found it difficult to breathe. She had heartburn and stomach pains, especially when something negative happened in the family or at work. She suffered from high levels of anxiety and was scared of almost any event that was not a part of her normal daily routine. On her back she had several moles that had appeared in adulthood and she was afraid that some of them might become cancerous.

At my request she also told me something about her psychological life. She was a highly punctual and ordered person who took pains to ensure that everything was as it should be. She loved singing, performed in public and took part in competitions, although on one occasion anxiety had caused her voice to falter and she had had difficulty keeping going. In her younger days she had played the piano. She loved dance, which, she said, seemed to her a more natural form of movement. She didn't like being completely alone; there had to be someone at home for her to feel secure. She felt anxiety. She suffered from self-pity. She avoided conflicts, she didn't know how to argue, she either broke into tears or backed down if she found herself in a conflict of interests. She then felt additionally aggravated by the way she had behaved and was angry with herself. She liked hiking and any type of trip to the country, including skiing. As a child, her father had beaten her frequently and often unjustly, and she feared him. She liked travelling, drove fast but safely and liked overtaking. She preferred holidaying in hot climates by the sea, where her problems improved and she felt generally better. But in the plane on the journey home the pains would return again with their original force.

In this case as well, the path to the selection of medicine was primarily psychological. The medicine should have the following characteristics: a highly unbalanced emotional state; up and down; traumatic damage in childhood as a result of parental violence; artistic tendencies (singing, piano playing) and a love of dance; a desire for perfection; fear of cancer; a great love of the countryside; weeps when she talks of her problems during the homeopathic interview; a high sensitivity to any disharmony (arguments, stress) or, on the other hand, harmony (love of the countryside, music) in her surroundings. Her case also demonstrated typical features of the remedy in relation to so-called "generals"—or the general character of the pathology—ailments improve by the sea and temporarily worsen in the early evening.

The medicine that I prescribed, and whose name I'll divulge in a while, is perhaps the most important for the worn-out syndrome as manifested sooner or later in people of this type. It is precisely that type of psychological and physical tiredness for which there is generally no explanation, even after the appropriate medical examinations. The fundamental psychological state of this type of person was very well described to me by a man who needed the same medicine for his ailments. He said: "I have the feeling that I'm an angel who, due to some minor misdemeanour, or rather out of curiosity, was born into this life on earth and who wants to be accepted and liked by the people around him. But somehow it doesn't quite work out for me, I keep coming up against problems and obstacles. This world is too rough for me, too immoral, too imperfect and wounding, as if I were still used to a higher order, existing in a heavenly realm; that's why I can't ever feel right here." The main subject of this medicine is seeking lost harmony.

I recommended *Carcinosin* (also known as *Carcinosinum*) 200C, a single tablet.

Carcinosin is a medicine whose holistic and especially mental picture was discovered in the nineteen-fifties, but which was only included in the Materia Medica and Repertory in the 1990s. At the time, many homeopaths such as the Australian Philip M. Bailey or the Frenchman J. Hui Bon Hoa announced that it was the most useful and most frequent constitutional type and medicine in their practice. I can only second their opinion. In my practice I have many instances of people who have been helped by *Carcinosin*, not only in mild or acute cases but also in long-lasting, chronic and sometimes very serious states, from flu, warts, arthrosis, allergies, eczema, colitis, migraine, to diabetes, anorexia, insomnia, phobias, depression and anxiety. It is interesting that the medicine's origin is unknown. All that is known is that the London-based Nelson's Pharmacy acquired it at the beginning of the nineteen-twenties from the USA in a 30C potency that was then further potentised. The original medicine can therefore not occur at lower than a 30C potency. It is not known from exactly what it is produced. The most likely explanation, however, is that it was developed by J.T. Kent, who removed and potentised the transparent, watery discharge from an open cancerous tumour in one of his patient's breasts and called it *Carcinosin*. On his own, however, Kent used it only for symptomatic purposes to reduce the pain of cancer sufferers, or to improve it, and was not aware of its wider application. A medicine produced from a person carries the vibration of the sick person, who feels and knows that his organism has been separated from the higher source and falls into disharmony and chaos.

Carcinosin falls under the category of so-called nosodes, i.e.

medicines made from pathological fluids, secretions etc. It is the only one of them, however, to contain no specific micro-organism and is exclusively the product of the human body; the only such medicine in homeopathy is *Lac humanum*, potentised human milk, at present a new medicine which has been little tested. It's no surprise that these two medicines have a very similar picture, or effect. Both come from the human breast, in the second case from a completely healthy breast. A point to consider: Why is it that a high percentage of homeopathic patients react holistically to the pure potentised product of the human body? (We'll find the answer in the second part of the book).

The woman with ankylosying spondylitis came for a follow-up on 19 April 2001, this time without ankylosying spondylitis. Her back had ceased to give her pain. Only in cold temperatures did she feel pain in the back region. The muscle cramp had passed. She was no longer tired. The pigmentation on her back had lightened in tone. Psychologically she felt far better, she smiled more, was more talkative, she felt less sorrowful, no longer had feelings of anxiety and didn't weep any more. Her wrist and toes continued to give her intermittent pain.

In June of the same year she had a two-day fever that passed on its own account. She felt fine. The pain in her wrist disappeared.

In September of the same year the pain and anxiety began to return. She again began to feel tired. What did this mean? A relapse, i.e. a return to the original pathology, although not yet to the state before treatment. I prescribed *Carcinosin* 1M.

In January 2002 she reported: three days after taking the medicine she felt extremely tired; on the fourth day the tiredness passed entirely and she began to feel extremely well psychologically. Her joints had given her discomfort for a few days, but what was that compared with her previous ailments?! At this point her development was entirely in accordance with Hering's first law, i.e., that symptoms must be treated from inside out. The deeper-seated pathology—tiredness and anxiety—disappears, while the surface symptoms—the joints—temporarily worsen. This provided an extremely positive prognosis for future development. This is exactly what happened: She began to feel calmer and more balanced and the pain in her joints gradually subsided. The back pain disappeared. Pigmentation on her skin, similar to that she had experienced after conventional medicines, appeared for a few hours. This means the manifestation of an old symptom, the temporary return of a state that she had experienced in the past, even though she was no longer taking any medicines. On the path upwards, therefore, she lived through previous frequency states which themselves had passed without the need for medicine. In April 2002, she again experienced mild back pain in cooler temperatures or when she sweated and suffered from repeated headaches. I recommended *Carcinosin* 50M.

In July 2002, she visited me because of her daughter. She didn't talk much about herself but started talking about something else altogether. She looked very happy and smiled constantly. Since previously she had often telephoned me if she had had problems it was safe to assume that she had not suffered anything worth mentioning.

I do not, however, want to pretend that all of my hundreds of cases of chronic illness were quite so clear-cut, nor, more importantly, that I was always successful from the outset in finding the resonating medicine that would cure and continue to act positively on the patient for many years, even if this has actually been the case in a significant percentage of my patients. This is not common in homeopathy and I have known quite highly-regarded homeopaths who have been unable to determine the action Hering's Laws in their cases. This means that they have not used precisely resonating medicines, or, more probably, that they have been unable to find them.

Finding the right medicine is demanding work that can

only be undertaken after an extensive interview. You have to process the relevant typical symptoms, by computer or in book-form, to decide on the right parts of the Repertory and to compare the probable remedies covering the symptoms with the patient and the Materia Medica. Sometimes it can be very difficult to decide between different medicines as all of them seem to correspond to the patient. At other times it seems that no medicine meets the relevant criteria. Whereas expert homeopathic journals and books are full of descriptions of cases where the resonating medicine was found quickly and smoothly, in private the authors will tell you that in their practice they have many cases where they change and try out a wide variety of medicines without a fundamental improvement in the patient's problems and only a temporary, mild amelioration (although in cases where conventional medicine has entirely failed the patients are obviously very happy for any relief). Or not even that. For example, before *Carcinosin* was introduced into holistic therapy, this was also the case with all those patients who today are successfully treated with this medicine. And other medicines are constantly being discovered. But even so, there are more than enough such prolonged and difficult cases. Sometimes it proves impossible to influence the overall decline in any way. Even the best homeopaths have such cases. The original picture of the patient's pathology, his fundamental vibrational pattern, may also be masked by previous or ongoing medication using chemical medicines and therefore might not appear on the surface in pure form, which makes it impossible to provide an accurate prescription that gets close to the centre's frequency. I will describe one such case which ultimately ended with the prescription of the correctly resonating medicine.

A patient was sent to me by a doctor whose child I had cured some years before. I had also helped other relations of his recover from quite long-standing problems. Probably this was why the patient retained her trust in me for so long, despite the problems refusing to go away. It was quite an extreme case and certainly not typical, but I describe it here because it portrays very well the stumbling blocks and twists and turns that we often have to confront on the path to a homeopathic holistic cure of ailments that have proved incurable by conventional treatment. It also shows a limit to homeopathy that we come up against not infrequently.

She arrived in January 2000, forty-five years old, well turned out, with a tense expression on her face. She told me a tale full of pain. For seven years she had suffered from severe migraines. The pain was on the left side of the head and during a migraine her neck would go numb. The head was also sensitive to touch. Her migraines lasted three days, despite her constantly taking pain-killing drugs. She used these preventively because the pills had no effect once the pain had begun. She structured the intensity of the pain from 1 to 5. The first level was already bad enough; the fifth level of pain was even resistant to injections.

The neurologist didn't know what to do with her. She usually suffered from the migraines once and sometimes twice a week. The pain had driven her to the edge of despair. Seven years before she had had cysts on her ovaries; these had been surgically removed along with her womb and ovaries. She had then undergone hormone replacement therapy and it was at this time that she had begun to suffer from migraines. She also suffered from insomnia, which likewise dated from the surgical removal of the womb and ovaries. She couldn't fall asleep without taking a sleeping pill, even if she waited more than two hours. Three times a year she had infections of the bladder. When she felt a sense of injustice she broke into tears. She liked company. She preferred to back down in an argument but not always; at work and at home she often defended her position. She liked walking in the country, and going to the forest to collect mushrooms; she was an avid reader, mainly of novels and thrillers. She sometimes rode a bicycle. She was superstitious and spat when ever she saw a cat. She had terrible dreams about war and a fear that her husband would leave her. She felt very anxious before a test. She had butterflies in the stomach before any event that didn't fit into her established routine. She felt the cold and liked to have a temperature of around 25^0 C in her house.

Of the general character of her complaints she said that they were worse in the morning, which generally began with a migraine. She also felt worse after an afternoon sleep. Her problems were exacerbated by low pressure and in cold, rainy weather. Some time before she had had a lump removed from her left breast. The operations had left behind protruding keloid scars. Since childhood she had suffered from constipation.

When I reflected on the character of her ailments, her own character and likes, with their emphasis on reading, and the disposition to keloid scars, I came to the conclusion that *Carcinosinum*, which contains these characteristics, would be the appropriate remedy, and I recommended a 200C potency, one dose. I was also led to this decision by the fact that by this time I had had several cases of chronic migraine which had been cured by the same medicine.

After one month she told me that the headaches had worsened. She now suffered them on a daily basis and nothing would help. None of the other ailments had shown any improvement. She still went to work, but this took up much of her energy. At this stage of her development I considered that the problem might be down to an unusually strong and prolonged "homeopathic aggravation", and that we should therefore wait to see how it would develop further. Two months later, however, her condition had still shown no improvement, which meant that the aggravation was not "homeopathic". She was taking pain-killers and sleeping pills.

Some time went by and her condition still didn't improve. Worse, she scalded her hand and had to stay at home for ten days. Experience tells me, although I can't generalise from it, that people under the effect of a precisely resonating medicine don't have serious accidents. An accident is not a coincidence and often is in some way mysteriously related to the psychological state of the person involved. So, in short, I had to find another homeopathic medicine. *Carcinosin* wasn't it. I finally decided on *Folliculinum*, a medicine produced from oestrogen, a component of the contraceptive pill. Interestingly, at the very start of her problems her head began to hurt and she began to suffer from insomnia immediately after she began to use hormone pills. Before losing her ovaries she had had various problems with ovulation. She fitted the medicine's main characteristic very well: problems suffered by people who try to hard to satisfy others. This could have been her case. There were many other reasons to choose *Folliculinum*, among them hot flushes. At the time I had just published a detailed description of *Folliculinum* in my homeopathic journal, and it struck me as a very promising medicine, even if new and little-tested in practice.

She took *Folliculinum* 200C. A few days later the migraines eased somewhat and she was again able to live without pain. Her sleeping also improved, although she was still dependent on pills to help her sleep. The improvement lasted several weeks and then everything began slowly to deteriorate again. Then, after she took another dose of the same medicine, she experienced over the course of five days a rapid deterioration that refused to improve. The medicine had only worked partially; a more precise resonance had not occurred. Her hot flushes got worse. She became very tearful.

I then tried *Sulphur* 200C. Again, there were many good reasons for prescribing it, such as the hot flushes, and the medicine also covered most of the other symptoms. *Sulphur* also has the reputation in complicated and over-prescribed cases of being able to remove the overlay of previous medications and of clarifying the original picture of the pathology, which homeopaths need in order to make a precise prescription.

Which is exactly what happened. The medicine may not have cured anything, but within a month of taking it she told me that she was by no means a domineering personality, and that consequently she never had arguments as she would always submit in any conflict; that she was extremely careful; that hot rooms made her feel uncomfortable, even though she was very sensitive to the cold; that she had always had a natural tendency to lose weight; and that she had never sweated, but now she sweated a lot, under the arms and on her forehead. In short, all of a sudden she was describing herself in quite different terms to those of a year before, when she had first come to see me. This time, thanks to *Sulphur*, it was a true picture of the person I was seeing, a picture of the original person, not repressed or altered by many years of using medication. Her description of herself immediately offered a logical whole. This was a picture of the remedy *Silica*.

After one pill of *Silica* 30C everything changed according to Hering's Laws of Cure. The very first day she had a severe headache and a stiff neck down to her back. The homeopathic aggravation had begun. She soon began to sleep without the help of a sleeping pill (for the first time in years). She still suffered headaches, but at ever longer intervals and not with the same intensity. The tearfulness disappeared at the very beginning. The old bladder problems reappeared and just as quickly disappeared. She was able to function normally both at work and at home. After three months she had no ailments whatsoever and likewise took no pills. After a few months of full health her sleeping worsened and she took Silica 200C. She said that she had perfect energy. The constipation she had suffered from for the whole of her life also passed. She ceased sweating excessively. She had taken several tests at work and for the first time in her life she was calm before them. She had gone a whole year without contracting flu, whereas previously she would catch it twice a year. She was a completely new person.

After half a year without any complaints she again began to suffer from mild headaches and insomnia. She was prescribed *Silica* 1M and returned to full health for another half-year. Then, before other tests, she again suffered from mild headaches and intermittent insomnia. I gave her *Silica* 10M. Everything returned to normal, although only for three months, after which the headaches returned, again intermittently. Every two weeks she had to take pain-killers and the insomnia reappeared; she would wake at three in the morning and be unable to get back to sleep. From a catastrophic situation to a full and long-lasting cure—but only temporary! Her frequency characteristic had changed and the medicine, originally accurate, had ceased to fit her case—a common enough event, even during flawless homeopathic therapy. The resonance was lost. I thus sent her away with the Autopathic Bottle and instruction on how to produce a highly-diluted autopathic preparation in a potency of 80C.

A month and a half after using the autopathic preparation she reported the following: her sleep had rapidly improved and she now slept perfectly. Her head had improved over the previous fortnight and only hurt if she drank alcohol at work (she had always been very sensitive to alcohol). This was from the centre outwards—a model reaction. It was just a shame that we hadn't known more about autopathy two years earlier.

Half a year earlier her husband had also visited me. He was a musician, with a variety of minor problems which all disappeared after *Carcinosin*. It was no coincidence that I had also considered *Carcinosin* for his wife. I have noticed that in the case of married couples (and life partners) we often find in homeopathic analyses a high occurrence of the same features and the same possible remedies. In short, they are in many things alike. Love itself is nothing other than a mutual resonance on a higher frequency level. If no resonance occurs, or it weakens, they will be indifferent to each other. The choice of

a partner, if love is the main criterion, is only the result of resonance with someone who is internally sufficiently similar to
oneself. Although it is never entirely the same—we also seek
qualities in our partner that are lacking in ourselves. Love at
first sight is a typical example of immediate resonance.

We generally desire a partner who is on a higher frequency
level than ourselves. Only in this way can they influence us
positively and not drag us down. As soon as the *Silica* had
allowed my patient to reach her higher frequency level she
helped her partner on the same path by bringing him to me
and to his constitutional medicine.

The above case is meant to show (which is typical for homeopathy) how long the search for the appropriate *simillimum*
can be, through a mass of other, sometimes partly-acting
medicines. In serious states, such as this one, a medicine that
resonates with the overall constitution, a *simillimum*, must
absolutely be found if the patient is really to be restored to
health. If this proves impossible (which sometimes happens
even despite the best efforts and skills) full health will not
be restored and the best that can be hoped for is a palliation
(which is also highly welcome) of the illness. For this to happen, however, a medicine must still be prescribed accurately,
i.e. through a deep knowledge of therapy and professional
tools such as the Repertory (more than a thousand pages)
or the computer repertory program and the Materia Medica
(a good homeopath always has several versions of the repertories and Materia Medica so as to be able to add and compare data). Imprecise or random prescriptions usually do not
result in resonance, or this is barely recognisable. Above all,
if there is resonance, for example during provings of medicines, it is very temporary. Ultimately, this case showed that
the effect of a homeopathic medicine, however precisely prescribed, may fade with time and that it may become necessary to move on.

The final homeopathic case that I want to describe here

concerns Karel, a company manager, forty years old and the father of two children. He first came to me six years ago complaining of pain in the frontal sinuses, headaches, bad flatulence after eating, chronic throat ache and back pain. He often woke in the night after terrible dreams and with the passing of time he was increasingly afflicted by feelings of fear. These paralysed him before a number of daily events, particularly tests and appearing in public, which was an unavoidable part of his job. He had suffered from all these problems for years. Conventional treatment hadn't been of much help and so he had visited a doctor who gave him various homeopathic medicines at the same time, without taking a detailed homeopathic case. This had had no effect either, and so he found his way to me.

Certain strong characteristics pointed clearly to *Lycopodium* —managerial type, aggravation of all ailments in the afternoon between five and eight o'clock, problems predominantly on the right side of the body, anxiety before appearing in public and before tests. I recommended *Lycopodium* 1M, a single dose. Shortly after taking it his headaches, the pain in his sinuses and throat ache ceased completely. Over the course of the first year his feelings of fear improved significantly and his nightmares passed. Satisfaction with the treatment lasted two years, with a single further prescription of *Lycopodium* 1M. Certain old ailments would sometimes appear for a few hours or days: stabbing stomach pains, an eczematic rash that lasted a couple of days, similar to one he had had in puberty.

After two years, due to continued anxiety about appearing in public, he took a higher potency, a higher dilution, of *Lycopodium*. This time it was *Lycopodium* 10M (diluted ten thousand times). Three years after commencing treatment he had had only one brief spell of influenza, and tests conducted by his brother, a doctor, showed that all blood, urine and other levels were absolutely normal, which they had not previously been. A model case, or so it seemed. Yet a year later his anxiety and fears began to rise again without explanation; they caused him to wake in the night, his sleep worsened, and he fell into depression. He also frequently began to feel cold and to shiver. His nose was permanently blocked. He tried the *Lycopodium* 10M again, this time without any result. *Carcinosin* was another medicine that homeopathically corresponded to the patient's picture. He took a 1M potency and the insomnia, which had had a debilitating effect, immediately disappeared. But it returned two months later and he could no longer be sure of sleeping. Other symptoms, particularly depression, also improved for a while, but refused to go away completely. After six months he was back to the former level of depression. He took *Carcinosin* 50M, but three months later he reported that there had been no major positive change—he slept fairly well but woke up sweating, stomach taut with fear, a sensation that lasted most of the day. He complained that it was unbearable.

From a homeopathic point of view the situation was quite common: the effect of one medicine had ended and the effect of a second was somewhat lower and was also wearing off. It was necessary to find something new. Every homeopath finds himself in the same situation quite regularly. Sometimes it works, sometimes it doesn't. I gave him the Autopathic Bottle with the user guide enclosed in the box. And told him to follow the instructions in dissolving his own saliva in fifteen litres of water to a potency of 600C and to use once.

He telephoned three months later and reported: Immediately after taking the autopathic preparation the fear had got even worse. He was nervous and depressed. Fortunately he was on holiday with his family at the time and so the week during which he suffered these effects generally passed without problems. His state of mind then calmed down over the next month. He stopped waking up in a sweat. The depression and fear disappeared. His sleep was excellent. All his chronic physical ailments passed off. For a couple of days he had flu symptoms and diarrhoea. The potentised substance from his own body had produced an even more perfect resonance than the substance from a woman living in the nineteenth century (*Carcinosin*) and from a plant (*Lycopodium*). He was very satisfied and asked me to prescribe autopathy for his wife, who suffered from some minor complaints and had hitherto reacted quite well to the medicine *Sepia*. Two months later she came to me and told me that her husband was still well. A year after using the autopathic preparation he visited me once again. For ten months he had experienced no ailments, but then, over the previous two months, the feelings of tiredness had returned. I recommended that he prepare and use an autopathic preparation in the 1500C potency, again using the special Autopathic Bottle. Since that time he has not contacted me once to complain of any problem.

When I talk about this family I have to complete the family portrait by mentioning the son, whom I also treat. Five years ago, his father brought him to see me as he was constantly suffering from colds, coughs and earache. After prescribing *Tilia europaea* 30C (Linden Tree), all his ailments disappeared and he now enjoys constant good health and resistance to illness. Recently, on my advice, his father gave him *Tilia* 1M. This is one of several cases in which I have successfully used *Tilia*. It is quite difficult to diagnose *Tilia* and people who react holistically and over a long period of time to potentised *Tilia* are quite rare. It is a so-called "small remedy", which in homeopathic terminology means the same as "rare". When I repeated this case to Dr. Shah from India, who was lecturing at our Homeopathic Academy in Prague, he was very surprised, particularly when I showed him the enormous tree from which the medicine is derived. He had thought that it was just a "small" and tender flower.

Part II.
AUTOPATHY

1. History

The birth of a new discipline never comes without antecedents. It is formed through the work of many people and the wisdom of generations. In establishing the basic precepts of homeopathy Hahnemann drew much from the Classical inheritance of the Greek physicians and medieval alchemists, as well as from the extensive European herbalist tradition. Autopathy's roots also reach far back into the past. The therapeutic holistic effects of a person's own urine, for example, were known in India long ago and were widely used in Ayurveda. European folk healers recommended a person's own urine in closing wounds. Healing by means of human secretions, however, only assumed its proper and most effective form when some American homeopaths in the nineteenth century began to use potentised, highly diluted human secretions on the principle of *equalia equalibus curantur*, "same cures same". They referred to this as "isopathy" and proceeded mostly from the opinion influenced by common medical practice, which focuses on diagnosis and the cure of localised illnesses. For example, the well-known homeopath and contributor to the Materia Medica, Adolph Lippe, in an article in *The Homeopathic Physician* (April 1884, p83) cites his colleague Dr. Lux, who said that "In accordance with this principle, all contagious diseases carry with them in the shape of their infectious matter their curative remedy". They potentised the diseased secretions, for example in the case of epidemics, and then administered them to patients with the same illness. Obviously, this bears a certain resemblance to vaccination. They called the process "isopathy".

Today, isopathy is used to treat, among other things, people whose health has suffered as a result of a certain type of vaccination. They are given the same vaccine, but this time homeopathically diluted. The potentised poison of a viper can be used isopathically to treat a viper's bite. Nevertheless, this understanding of isopathy has certain drawbacks—it ignores certain central aspects of homeopathy, primarily its holistic concept. And it goes against what Hahnemann said about homeopathy: that it is treatment on the principle of "like cures like". Isopathy thus ceases to be homeopathy. Opinions on this matter, however, varied. In *The Medical Advance*, vol. XXXII, no. 2, 1894, p. 59, the well-known homeopathic doctor J.H. Allen of Indiana wrote: "I will give proof that I think will be fully convincing to most minds that so-called Isopathy is but the highest phase of *similia* in the highest sense."

The medications created on the basis of this philosophy were called nosodes. One of these nosodes, originally used to treat innate dispositions to cancer and to relieve pain caused by cancer was *Carcinosin*, which was prepared by J.T. Kent. Its full picture, enabling it to treat the whole organism, was discovered fifty years later.

Only in the twentieth century do we find the first instances of homeopaths daring to administer a potentised preparation to the same person from whom the pathological material was obtained. The classical French homeopath O.A. Julian has left a record of this in his book *Materia Merdica of the Nosodes*. He writes that he was on holiday when he was called to treat a man with very bad herpes and found himself (as he explains apologetically) without any remedies. "The herpes was on the left side of the face. Blisters and ulcers had spread to his forehead, face, cheek and upper lip; the mucous membrane of his left nostril and the upper part of the roof of the mouth had also been affected, as had a swollen left eyelid with blisters and swollen conjunctiva." He had a temperature of 38.8⁰ C and a quickened pulse. He suffered from insomnia, vomiting and strong headaches. Dr. Julian prepared an isopathic remedy from the discharge of an ulcer on the roof of his mouth. He diluted this in water to the sixth centesimal (a very low) potency, and mixed the final dilution with spirits. He then administered this preparation every half hour. To begin with the pain increased, but on the second day it fell markedly, the vomiting passed and the patient was able to sleep properly again. By the second day the herpes had already reduced by a half and the swelling had disappeared. Within a few days all that was left were some healthily falling scabs.

Nevertheless, I should say that references to isopathy or even autoisopathy (treatment of the same person from whom the material was obtained) are extremely rare in homeopathic literature. In my computer I have the ReferenceWorks homeopathic programe, which contains many materia medicas and repertories, some of them ten volumes long, plus thousands of pages of articles from specialist magazines, yet if I use the search engine to find these and related words from among the entire volume of the literature it only comes up with a few, very brief references. The example cited above is the only well-described case of auto-isopathic treatment that I have been able to find in the vast library of ReferenceWorks. And this was not even a holistic treatment.

Of particular interest is the reference by the French doctor Hui Bon Hoa in an article on *Carcinosin* for the *British Homoeopathic Journal*. His note is a single sentence, which for this subject is quite typical: "Some patients who have responded to *Carcinosin* but whose improvement only lasted a short time have derived benefit from auto-isopathy. I give a single dose of Pharyngeal Mucus 30CH." A sentence that, if we think about it, merits expanding into a thick and sizeable book that could bring much relief to the sick. It points out that potentised, ordinary, non-pathological phlegm from one's own body can have a holistic effect on the health of most people that use it. It is, however, just a fragmentary reference and there is nothing more on this method in the article.

This and similar references nevertheless arouse one's curiosity. Thus, some years ago, I began to look into the subject more deeply. For example, in an old catalogue from an English homeopathic pharmacy, I found an offer to produce a high potency of a person's own blood or other bodily fluids. When I asked if they could give me these potencies they replied that they could not continue this line. They did not explain why. One of the pharmacy's employees did, however, inform me that they had produced these preparations and they had many years' experience with them, particularly with animals. And that for such a treatment it was necessary to go up to a very high potency. He wrote to me: "the higher the better." That such treatment is regularly practised on animals in England is testified to by the reference (again brief) in Dr. MacLeod's *Veterinary Homeopathy* (C. W. Daniel, 2000).

The result of these researches was the discovery that auto-isopathy is a sort of thirteenth chamber of homeopathy. And there followed an irrevocable decision—to continue in this line. To gather information and experience. To take steps to make it possible to potentise a person's own fluids, these being healthy, normal saliva (without abnormal admixtures of pathogenic bacteria or viruses) which are undoubtedly "…the highest phase of *similia* in the highest sense" and carry detailed information of the state of the whole organism. As was to be shown later, they really are capable of being most precisely tuned to the frequency of the fine-matter creative centre inside the person of which they are the material product. Elevated by potentisation in pure water into homeopathic dilution—the fine-matter form—they can, using a precise resonance, cause the sick person's enfeebled fine-matter creative sphere (the dynamis) to reverberate again in its original frequency and bring about a return to the organism's original structure; to health. It is no longer a matter of the highest and nearest similarity of the healing product, but directly of sameness; of the nearest frequency structure that may occur in nature. The closest similarity is sameness.

2. Why "Autopathy"?

I should finally explain why I call it "autopathy" and not "isopathy", or "autoisopathy". The term is not my invention, it comes from the British Homoeopathic Library's list of professional terms published on its website, where autopathy is mentioned as one of the terms under autoisopathy. As is evident above, the word "isopathy" is closely related to the treatment of localised pathology. The discharge of a certain illness cures this same illness. Isopathy has thus historically not claimed to be a holistic form of treatment. This book, however, deals exclusively with a holistic approach, in the spirit of Hahnemann's well known idea: "I don't cure the illness, but the person". That is why I have chosen a term that is not encumbered by this "pathological" consideration. And because it is totally new, neither is it encumbered by a mass of other prejudices that have sometimes originated in homeopathy as part of the numerous "schools" and approaches. Autopathy does not seek a *simillimum*—a similar medicine—and it does not use homeopathic medicines. But it has philosophical and historical roots in homeopathy, as well as in the teachings of Buddha, Swedenborg, Kabbalistic rabbis, Indian or Celtic shamans, yogis, and the beliefs of the early Christians, Rosicrucians, Sufis, people practising channelling (mental communication with higher dimensions) and many others. Autopathy, enriched from different sources, is a continuation of homeopathy by other means. I understand it primarily as a spiritual discipline, an individual journey to connect with the higher levels of the universe. Improving the organisational function of the individual higher creative sphere leads necessarily to an improvement in the person's entire hierarchical spiritual system, throughout his physical body and onwards. A person who is healing spiritually extends his high vibrations throughout his whole environment; in his family and his community he is able to improve the lives of similarly tuned people. Autopathy is a means by which to establish overall harmony. It is a gradual homeopathic journey to a state of higher understanding and happiness.

3. How to Obtain an Autopathic Preparation

In order to practise autopathy we need an autopathic preparation. Once we have this we can gain experience, experiment and above all cure. At present, however, only a few production facilities exist in Europe that are able to prepare an autopathic preparation from a person's own bodily fluid. The technology of potentising a patient's bodily fluids in such a facility would anyway raise certain problems. The fluid has to be transported across large distances and mixed with spirits in order to prevent it from "spoiling" during the journey—the effect of bacteria on its frequency structure, which is the imprint of the entire organism's frequency structure. This obviously comes at a price, with the fluid's qualities anyway being altered through the admixture of alcohol. It is known that alcohol has its own homeopathic (frequency) pattern, which anyone who has ever drunk too much is well aware of. A mixture of two patterns is thus created in which, nevertheless, the patient's imprint plays the decisive role. We could say the same about mixing with lactose (a sugar), which is sometimes used instead of alcoholic spirits. In a pharmacy, or more precisely a pharmaceutical production point, the fluid mixed with alcohol is potentised in dilution machines, which are usually powered by electricity when succussing (shaking) the flask. This means that a magnetic field is created during production which may also influence the preparation's frequency qualities. As a result, it may be that the subsequent preparation is only "similar", or a *simillimum*, partly resonating but not the "same", not fully resonating. The pharmaceutical production process makes it wholly impossible to produce a medicine for acute needs, quickly and for immediate use; for example, in the case of an acute illness or sudden relapse, if a prior dose suddenly ceases to have effect. People currently have practically no opportunity to use an auto(iso)pathic preparation, or at least to try one. My first thought, therefore, when I discovered that there was something in autopathy, was somehow to organise the means for the quick and straightforward production of a high potency directly in the home, and to bypass the laboratory entirely. I first studied the history of potentising, of which I obviously already had some knowledge. I found a wealth of detail on the subject in Julian Winston's excellent history of homeopathy (*The Faces of Homeopathy*, Great Auk Publishing, 1999).

For most of his life, the discoverer of homeopathy potentised medicines by placing a plant tincture, for example, in a glass vial, the tincture amounting to one-hundredth of the vial's volume. He then added 99 parts of distilled water. He shook this with strong succussions on a firm, elastic base (usually a book). He transferred one hundredth of the contents of the first vial to a new, clean, as yet unused vial and poured in 99 parts of distilled water before shaking again. And so on, thirty, even two hundred times. He thus came by a two hundred centesimal dilution, 200C. This method placed great demands on the consumption of glass. Hahnemann found that a vial that was completely and reliably emptied of the potentised liquid retained the potency and was capable of transferring it. This "memory of the glass" means that no one vial can be used to produce two medicines as this would lead to their "cross-contamination", to their mixing, and thus the invalidation of the preparation. At the end of his life he started to produce the preparations by another means, which is described in the sixth, and final, edition of the *Organon*. The process is exceptionally demanding and complex and is suitable only for the laboratory. Medicines produced in this manner are nowadays called LM or Q potencies and are still used.

Later, when a demand for high potencies arose, medicines began to be produced on potentising machines. The American homeopath Dr. Dunham used to fasten flasks to a steam hammer to ensure they were shaken as strongly as possible.

/79

In general, however, it became clear that a medicine's effect increased the more it was diluted, sometimes up to thousands and tens of thousands of times and even beyond.

In the second half of the nineteenth century, Dr. Thomas Skinner (1825–1926) put forward the theory that vigorous shaking was not such an important part of the preparation, and that it basically only helped ensure a thorough mix of the liquid, which could also be done in different ways. Skinner's machine was the first flux equipment for the production of homeopathic potencies. This was used in the American pharmacy of Boericke & Tafel for a hundred and thirty years. Skinner's machine contained two vials revolving along a transverse axis with the neck moving upwards and downwards. These were filled firstly with a tincture of the substance, then water, then emptied and refilled with water, emptied again and refilled... The drops that remained on the walls of the vials represented roughly one-hundredth of the volume and transferred the potency to another filling. This was the flux of the water. Through his machine Skinner achieved dilutions that corresponded to one hundred thousand Hahnemann centesimal dilutions. Most homeopathic medicines above 1M (1000C), including those administered by the most famous and most successful American, English and Indian homeopaths during the twentieth century, were produced by this machine. Its importance, at least for homeopaths and their patients, is indisputable.

Dr. Bernhardt Maximilian Fincke (1821–1906) of New York arrived at a similar idea. He first achieved a potency of 6C or 30C by diluting in alcohol, then, in his own laboratory, introduced water from the New York water system (!) into the flask with spirit potency of 30C and allowed it to flow through very slowly for varying periods, an hour or a day or several days. In those days, the water from the water system evidently did not contain chemical admixtures. In this way he achieved dilutions comparable with Hahnemann's 1M (one thousand potency), 10M (ten thousand potency), 50M (fifty thousand potency) and CM (one hundred thousand potency). J.T. Kent was one of many to use Fincke's medicines, and wrote of them that they acted quickly, lastingly and deeply. Indeed, so highly was Fincke regarded for his work concerning the flux production of potentised preparations that in 1896 he was elected president of the International Hahnemannian Association. Over time, however, his efforts have largely been forgotten and many contemporary practitioners do not even know his name. Nevertheless, the flux method is still sometimes used to prepare medicines today, including in the laboratories of well-known producers.

Homeopathy also knows another method, known as the Korsakov[3] dilution, which has been used for more than a hundred and fifty years and which may have influenced the invention of Skinner's machine. One hundredth of the tincture of the substance to be potentised (e.g. a drop) is placed inside a flask. The diluting agent, water or alcoholic spirit, is then poured into it. After the flask has been filled it is emptied of the entire contents. Sometimes the flask is succussed, sometimes not. The effect is the same. The flask is then filled again, emptied and refilled with the diluting agent, emptied and so on. The drops on the walls of the flask transfer information from one refill to the next. This type of dilution is considered to be comparable with the Hahnemann centesimal dilution. Production facilities sometimes use electric power to succuss the flask, fill and empty it. Thirty refills mean a potency of 30C.

The experience of many generations of homeopaths, together with my own practice, has led me to realise that the last two procedures are the most suitable for the reliable preparation of autopathic medicines in the home. Later, I will look

---

[3]   Semyen Korsakov—Russian homeopath and nobleman (1788–1853), inventor of the special method of potentisation. He was also the first man who potentised human blood.

in more detail at their practical preparation in this environment.

4. Bodily Fluids

Every one of our bodily fluids bears a frequency structure that is identical to the frequency structure of the organism as a whole, and to the frequency structure of our fine-matter creative system, which is many octaves higher. As we have already remarked, the fine-matter system consistently organises all events in our material body. If its creative frequency weakens or changes into a lower frequency, we will fall ill. If our higher creative sphere reverberates through resonance with a potentised bodily fluid from our own body the organism's original structure will return—the original health that we enjoyed before we fell ill.

Autopathy believes in using the healthiest bodily fluid to produce a potentised preparation. Such a fluid is the most reliable carrier of the overall organism's frequency structure. An infected fluid full of bacteria (pus etc.) will not properly correspond to the state of the fine-matter sphere because it contains a large quantity of other organisms. This approach distinguishes autopathy from isopathy, which often uses pathologically changed discharges, secretions or heavily diseased tissues to produce potencies.

In the past, isopathy was also associated with a symptom-based approach—it was often mentioned as a treatment for a specific illness or ailments. Autopathy, on the other hand, is unquestionably a holistic therapy. Every part of the organism and every bodily fluid carries complete information about the whole, or about the individual frequency structure of the person's higher organisational sphere. The less the bodily fluid is directly affected by disease or another disorder, the better it will carry information about the overall state of the organism, including the relevant disease or ailment. And it will more faithfully retain the essential frequency structure. For example: A person is suffering from an inflamed bladder with a high incidence of bacteria in his urine. An isopathic approach would certainly consider potentising the infected urine. In autopathy, however, we would definitely favour using saliva, which, unlike the urine, will not have any abnormal bacterial content. This will better tune the organism back to health and cure the inflamed bladder.

For potentising purposes it is basically possible to use any fresh, relatively healthy bodily fluid as an initial substance. Every fluid that comes from a person's body carries information about the entire organism's frequency. Not, however, always to the same extent.

In the past, the auto-isopathic treatment of chronic and acute illness recorded positive results with preparations from the subject's own blood, both for animals and people. Today, however, for reasons of hygiene, **blood** is closely monitored by the authorities and all procedures with it are subject to strict regulations. Neither is it ideal from the point of view of its function:

a) In order to obtain blood, it is necessary to break the skin. This is painful and in certain circumstances the wound may become infected. More importantly, however, the process of drawing blood causes trauma, the vibrations of which affect the entire organism and leave traces in the vibrational structure of the blood. The acute trauma slightly alters the information on the organism. We prefer to obtain, if possible, an unaltered, current frequency picture of the relevant person.

b) Immediately after leaving the vascular system the blood alters; it coagulates. Blood on the skin's surface or in a hypodermic syringe is not the same as the blood that circulates inside the body.

c) The blood may be changed by disinfecting the skin before it is punctured. For example, if iodine tincture is used, traces may get into the blood. Nevertheless, a woman attending the Homeopathic Academy did tell me that her daughter's chronic eczema had markedly improved after she gave her repeated doses of her own blood potentised at the low potency of 6C.

Urine leaves the body entirely naturally and, like all other bodily fluids, bears the frequency structure of the entire organism. As it is produced in the lower part of the body and disposes of waste substances, its frequency characteristic is closer to the lowest chakras. We have already mentioned the long tradition associated with the use of a person's own urine in treating chronic illnesses. Many books have been published on urinotherapy. The daily use of one's own, undiluted urine is generally recommended, with effects ranging from the cure of serious illnesses, prolongation of life and the boosting of the immune system.

Indeed, my first—successful—experience with autopathy came with the potentising of urine.

There are also **other bodily fluids**—pure *phlegm* from the nasal and laryngeal cavities, *mother's milk, sperm, sweat* and *tears*. All carry frequency information about the entire organism and thus are capable, following homeopathic dilution, of treating holistically the person from whom they derived, regardless of the localisation or character of the problems. In his lecture on bowel nosodes given at the Academy of Homeopathy in Prague in May 2002, Dr. Russell Malcolm of the Faculty of Homoeopathy in London referred to English doctors who prescribe patients their own, highly (infinitesimally) diluted stool.

Saliva comes from areas that are closest to the most important chakras, transferring the creative frequency from the higher levels to our mind and physical organism. Their structure precisely reflects every occurrence in the organism as well as in the higher frequency levels (Hahnemann's *dynamis*, Kent's Inner Man) that are vital to the organism's very existence (whatever its state). An error in the higher hierarchic frequency levels causes illness in the physical organism—which is why it is precisely here, at the point of origin, that it must be remedied. The remedy must be the most closely resonating highly potentised substance. When I progressed from urine-based preparations to those prepared from saliva, I noticed a deeper reaction and a more striking holistic therapeutic effect. At present, I strongly recommend the use of a person's own saliva.

5. Method

An autopathic preparation essentially works in the same way as a precisely selected homeopathic constitutional medicine, prescribed according to an aggregate of the patient's symptoms. Consequently, autopathy also follows the vast majority of rules and principles established by Samuel Hahnemann, J.T. Kent, Constantine Hering, J.H. Clarke, Elizabeth Wright-Hubbard, George Vithoulkas and other well-known homeopaths.

A single dose

As a rule, I recommend that all potencies of 20C and above be taken only once. These should be administered immediately following their production. A few drops are sufficient. We must, however, be certain that these really do fall on the mucous membrane of the mouth (I will give detailed instructions on producing the preparation later). The length of time that a single dose will act on the organism depends primarily on the level of the potency (the amount of water used for the dilution) and the individual state of the organism. The higher the potency, the longer it will act (except very high potencies over 5M where it was not true in some cases). When using 40C in the case of chronic illness this generally means for at least three months, although sometimes many months longer, during which period the patient remains under the positive harmonising influence of the preparation. Each dilution extends the period of influence. In very old people a low potency diluted with a small quantity of water (half a litre in an Autopathic Bottle or twenty Korsakov dilutions) will act for a long time. In order to determine the point at which its effect starts to weaken or disappear we follow Hering's Laws, which have been applied in homeopathic treatment for over a hundred years. This enables us to maintain the results of treatment achieved thus far, or, where necessary, to move it on to another stage.

Laws of cure

I have already mentioned these, but given their importance and the fact that for most people they provide a rare insight into health and illness, it is worth dealing with them in a little more depth.

First to be affected by the preparation is the patient's higher, creative sphere. From here the therapeutic wave expands through the mind and emotions to the physical organs, also hierarchically, from the heart at the centre through the internal organs to the skin and the mucous membrane of the nose. The therapeutic wave thus proceeds *from within outward*—which is Hering's first law.

The therapeutic current is contrary to the natural process of declining health as we commonly experience it through the course of our life. Typical declining health begins in childhood with colds, then coughs, followed by inflammations of the bronchial tubes, asthma in adolescence and finally perhaps also depression. Pathology gradually proceeds from the periphery, for example from the mucous membrane of the nose, to the internal sphere (acute inflammation of the bronchial tubes), before settling in a chronic and life-threatening condition (bronchial asthma) which is exacerbated by heart problems and which ultimately also affects an even more internal sphere—the psyche (depression). With some people, this process can take place very rapidly or may even occur at a pre-natal stage. As soon as there is therapeutic resonance, the process described under Hering's **first law**, *from within outward*, can begin. The psyche is the first area to be cured with the relief of depression. Only then can the process of healing the cardiac ailments begin, and after that, the asthma. The curing of asthma may be accompanied by temporary inflammation of the bronchial tubes and the therapy concludes with colds, which formerly preceded the onset of more serious pathologies. We will understand this better if we imagine the previously mentioned staircase of health (see page 49).

After taking the autopathic preparation the patient will gradually pass through previous frequency states and through these the organism will return to the state of health it had at the beginning, or even further, to the original healthy frequency of Man; to the frequency archetype, located extremely high in the creative sphere. The return to health follows the same path as the descent into illness, although travelling in the opposite direction. Ailments may thus occur that existed in the past but are no longer (e.g. inflammation of the bronchial tubes). These will pass relatively quickly. I call them *reverse symptoms*. In his *Lectures on Homoeopathic Philosophy*, Kent referred to these symptoms thus: "Only a fool would regret the reappearance of old symptoms as they are the only way to recovery."

In reality, by no means all previous ailments reappear during the tuning stage. Some occur almost unnoticed, merely as an impression, perhaps just for an hour, or a day, as a fleeting sensation. But some can be more pronounced. These soon recede with the ongoing tuning of the organism to its original state. Months and later even years may pass between outbreaks. They can be treated conventionally or otherwise according to one's own judgement and their development. Conventional symptomatic treatment has no great effect on long-term general development. An old pain in the wrist or a fever may recur, usually for one or two days, flu symptoms, upset stomach and so on. For example, if someone suffered repeated sore throats three times a year, after taking the preparation the reverse sore throat will occur only once in a milder form. This also generally passes quickly.

It is always the case, however, that the organism begins to

improve immediately upon taking the preparation as the frequency of the creative sphere increases. For example: the first symptoms to disappear are depression and anxiety, the most deeply-located problems; these are followed by an amelioration of heart conditions and subsequently breathing problems associated with bronchial asthma. A deep cough then appears, passes and perhaps gives way to a cold. Throughout this period the person's health is being restored and the sense of ease with life increases. Hering's **second law** illustrates this process very nicely—*symptoms are cured in the opposite sequence to that in which they occurred.*

We know that feelings, like physical ailments, fluctuate during the day depending on the external environment and internal events. Over the course of the treatment, these fluctuations are directed upwards, to a greater feeling of comfort. Or, in the absence of a medicine resonating with the fine-matter centre, downwards, to ever more serious problems, to deeper pathology and greater suffering.

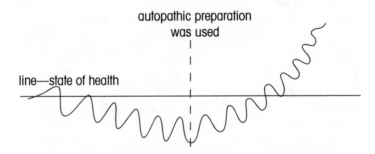

Fluctuations in health before and after taking the autopathic preparation. The state of health deteriorates. After taking the preparation it gradually improves.

Finally, Hering's **third law**—symptoms dispersed throughout the body are cured from above downwards. Originally it was the second law but I put it in the third place because of its lower importance than the previous two. This process is particularly evident for dermatological problems or, for example, in the case of pain in the joints. Sometimes I saw disruption of this law in otherwise successful cases. But this clearly derives from the process of healing from the centre; first to be healed are problems in the head, the centre, and then further down. It often happens that in cases of eczema the complaint disappears first from the hair and face before receding from the lower parts of the body. So, if a patient comes to us with eczema and complains that although the eczema has disappeared from her face it has got worse on her legs, we will know for sure that things are developing in the right direction. The treatment is continuing to work and just as the eczema disappeared from the face, so in time will it disappear from her legs without our having to intervene. We can explain the matter to the patient and give her that confidence.

After many years of practice I suggest the addition of two other rules:

The other (fourth) law (already not Hering's but in accordance with him) is that symptoms are healed in the order of their importance. The priorities are always set by the organism itself and I was sometimes surprised that it could in very rare cases break even Hering's Laws. For instance severe pains in hips (which were also limiting the person socially) disappeared sooner than minor problems with liver.

Healing crises appear at some time during the process of harmonisation. It means that almost every chronic problem worsens a little just before it is completely healed, even many months after taking the preparation. This is the **fifth law**.

Follow-ups during the treatment phase enable us to compare the case's development with the laws and thus to spot a potential relapse, a recurrence of symptoms that have already receded in time. Over time, the effect of the initial autopathic preparation may fade and disappear and the organism begin to return to its original pathology, its condition before treatment. It is important to identify this as soon as possible in order to prevent the recurrence of all the previously-removed ailments and to administer an autopathic preparation, usually of a higher potency, that will ensure the return to health continues and immediately put a halt to the deterioration.

In addition to monitoring the case according to laws, it is also essential to be able to perceive the so-called *homeopathic,* in our case *autopathic, aggravation.* This may, although not necessarily, occur in the first few hours, days and sometimes weeks following the initial dose of the resonating potentised preparation. Some ailments may temporarily worsen slightly after the preparation has been administered. In this respect, homeopathy speaks of internal therapeutic intelligence. In autopathy, as in homeopathy, aggravation after the initial dose may be considered a positive sign, showing that resonance has occurred. Aggravation can augur well for future improvement and the disappearance of the ailments. It is usually mild and brief. Indeed, in the majority of cases it is hardly noticeable. Moreover, because the potentised preparation acts hierarchically, our internal, fine-matter (spiritual) system is already healthier, meaning that we feel better in ourselves, even in the event of aggravation. Nevertheless, we should always pay proper attention to the possibility of aggravation occurring.

If an exceptional case of aggravation was felt to be more serious, or where there is doubt, it is obviously possible to regulate it through appropriate specialist care. The same is true in cases of the reappearance of old, reverse symptoms. Autopathy acts in a dimension above material medicines; it does not limit their effect and is not markedly limited by them—development continues. Only homeopathic medicines in high potencies have in some cases been able to antidote or stop the autopathic process. In classical homeopathy we use the rule that only one potentised substance can act (and be used) in one time. Administration of another potentised substance means a change of influence.

From a more general, philosophical point of view, autopathy is not used to cure illness. It is a means to increase the vibrations of a person's spiritual, creative sphere. It can gradually introduce harmony into your life, but always depending on your internal, individual, karmic disposition, which can differ from one person to another. Anyone who uses autopathy should be aware that he is working with something unknown, complex and indeterminable, with Man. Something can surprise you at any turn and, unlike in other types of treatment, one should never take anything for granted. Autopathy is a path, the complicated journey of life itself.

Purifying the organism

Especially in the first weeks after using the preparation, but generally at any point during treatment, certain mild reactions of a purifying character may occur in the organism. This may mean more frequent urination, more frequent stools or diarrhoea, increased sweating, colds and vaginal discharges. Waste substances generally are emitted in a higher measure. After these have disappeared (whether through using conventional medicines or otherwise) the patient will feel better than before. Other ways in which the pathological dissonance may be purged or discharged are through rashes, pimples etc. Aches in the joints may also be noticed. For example: insomnia and depression passed (these are internally located problems) but mild pain was felt in the knuckles (peripheral). These pass with time. Fever is also a reaction with a healing purpose; it testifies to the organism's increased activity and is a manifestation of its attempt to dispose of the pathology. In autopathy a fever of this kind generally lasts one day; the second day it tends to weaken or disappear altogether. So far, I have only encountered two cases in adults where the fever has lasted longer. Interestingly, in cases of fever of this sort, which occur rarely or only once, the patient usually feels quite well, does not lose energy and sometimes feels as if nothing is wrong with him. One woman, for example, went to work for several days with a very high temperature. After this she felt cleansed. I would not advise anyone to emulate her; she acted according to her choice. It would be better to rest. If complications arise and you feel discomfort it is always safer to seek medical help.

Making sense of these simple rules is not difficult, even if at the beginning they may be unfamiliar to people who are not used to holistic treatment. The processes in the organism that I describe above are not caused by diluted saliva! They are generated by the person's non-material, creative sphere. It is life itself.

6. What Are We Healing?

Equipped with the basic know-how, we can now begin to talk about the practical approach to treatment. It is exclusively the spiritual level that is healed and influenced by the non-material potency. The lower levels only testify to its condition and are one hundred per cent dependent on it. We do not heal illness but the inner Man, the non-material spiritual principle. The positively affected high, fine-matter sphere may, depending on the individual's personal inner karma[4], completely improve the person's system as a whole, from the spiritual state to a comprehensive physical cure, or gradually expand its influence to the social sphere and personal relations. Nonetheless, anyone who is not entirely familiar with the holistic concept of healing will probably ask what precisely autopathy is for, or where and for what sorts of ailments autopathy can get the best results.

My own experience is as follows: the list of chronic (in the terminology of conventional medicine meaning approximately the same as incurable) ailments that have radically improved or disappeared after autopathy is roughly the following and continues to grow (the diagnoses obviously aren't mine but rather those of the doctors whom my patients had previously visited without any marked success): chronic eczema, bronchial asthma, frequent or permanent headaches, chronic fatigue syndrome, insomnia, allergies, anxiety and depression, constant melancholy for no obvious reason, unaccountable fear, chronic coughs and repeated inflammation of the bronchial tubes, chronic colds, tearfulness and insomnia in babies, liver problems, ischaemic heart disease and associ-

---

[4]   *Karma* is a term used in Buddhism to describe the internal, spiritual and derived physical or social condition of man; based on his past thoughts and actions it is the result of his own conscious behavioural choices, not only in this life but in a number of previous lives.

ated problems, persistent metrorrhagia and associated tiredness, chronic inflammation of the intestines, pain and dysfunction of the gall-bladder, painful menstruation, high blood pressure, heart pains during physical exertion, constant rapid pulse, irregular and intermittent pulse, cramps in the legs, diabetes, diarrhoea, inflamed toenails, frequent vomiting in babies, digestive problems, pains in the joints, susceptibility to infectious diseases such as influenza and throat ache, lowered immunity and others.

I would like at this point to emphasise the old homeopathic truth that there are highly advanced pathological states in which a return to health is no longer possible. This is not a matter of types of illness but of the organism's overall vitality. If this is already weak it will not have sufficient strength to heal the organism. Sometimes we are not able to recognise this in a patient (age is not the main criterion here). We have to be humble. A person's karma, his inner state, is sometimes deeply concealed. Even in such cases, however, autopathy may bring at least some improvement in the quality of life, increased enjoyment, an improvement in the higher spiritual sphere, despite the lower material structures being incurable for the creative sphere.

Acute problems also recede rapidly following the administering of an autopathic preparation. I recommended an autopathic preparation to a young man who for several days had been suffering from a watery stool, a temperature ranging during the day from 37.6 to 39^0 C and who felt poorly and rather melancholic. He followed my instructions and created and used a 160C potency of his own saliva—the following day the problems had disappeared and his stool was back to normal. Since then he has been completely healthy for several months. This is not the only instance of fever receding rapidly after using autopathy. Be careful, however: this is not to suggest that in acute cases you should only rely on autopathy. It can also be used as a complementary method. Ultimately, the decision on the type and means of therapy always belongs to the patient.

I feel I should re-emphasise that acute illness, like chronic and long-term illnesses, is merely the result of a chronic disposition to illness, or miasm. According to the frequency theory, both acute and chronic illnesses are caused by a decrease in the frequency of the creative, organisational sphere, which is no longer able to preserve harmony—the original healthy structure, the healthy operation of the physical organism. The administering of an autopathic preparation in fine-matter form causes the centre to reverberate once again and renews the healthy structure of the hierarchically arranged physical organs.

We can of course assume that the young man's stool contained an excess of pathogenic micro-organisms. These, however, had disappeared by the next day as in a healthy intestine they are unable to find conditions in which to multiply or live off. Pathogenic micro-organisms are usually to be found in small amounts in every healthy organism. They begin to multiply abnormally when the organism loses its original structure (or health) through a fall in the fine-matter frequency. If the organism loses its internal fine-matter vitality it becomes a welcome source of sustenance for micro-organisms; if it loses its vitality entirely, it dies and the bacteria take over completely. An internally healthy organism, whose creative sphere is at its original high frequency, thus creating harmony in the physical organs, cannot be threatened by infection. During an epidemic we breathe the same air, meet the same people and eat the same food or drink the same water, but only some of us fall ill, even though everyone came into contact with the virus or bacteria. The reason is that some of us do not have a disposition towards illness due to the positive state of our creative centre. Others do have a disposition towards illness because their central frequency is low and thus unable to

/97

preserve the organism's harmony intact when faced with the onslaught from outside—thus they fall ill.

It is interesting that, in the past, terrible epidemics always occurred after catastrophic events that negatively affected the entire fine-matter sphere—including the mind. After wars, when people were demoralised by the killing, the loss of ideals, aggression and uncertainty and were destroyed by grief, when the "low-frequency" or "hellish" currents in society and the minds of men prevailed and significantly reduced people's individual frequencies. These currents drew attention to phenomena at the lowest ethical levels, when spiritual pathology prevailed. Examples include the typhoid epidemic in Leipzig after the Napoleonic Wars, the AIDS epidemic in Africa, where traditional ethical values are in the process of being completely destroyed, and the flu epidemic after the First World War, which killed ten million people in Europe and was coterminous with the birth of Fascist and Communist dictatorship. It was a time when the European and American populations retreated en masse from high religious ideals, a time of rising atheism, an exclusive interest in the economy and the purely material sphere. Homeopathy, which had hitherto recorded strong progress, almost died out at this time and was only reborn in the nineteen-eighties and nineties with the advance in holistic and ecological thinking.

Prevention

The successful *prevention* of a decline in health (in the context of the methods described) thus depends on the timely use of an autopathic preparation in a relatively healthy state and in an increase in the harmony of the entire organism, firstly at the highest fine-matter level. The principle is well-known from homeopathy, where, if a holistically-acting, highly-resonating constitutional medicine can be found, the patient's health will be strengthened profoundly and lastingly, and physical and psychological resistance will be increased. This is true for both children and adults. In my practice I have often noticed that children who were once repeatedly absent from school enjoy far higher levels of attendance and health after using autopathy. It is highly beneficial to use a high-potency autopathic preparation before the illness fully takes hold, when problems are still slight, superficial or occasional and can be easily and swiftly remedied. It is also highly recommended to use a preparation before entering a stressful or infectious environment. People who enjoy full health will also feel tangible benefits. In particular people who are seeking closer contact with the higher creative sphere, whether through meditation, channelling, shamanic techniques, prayer etc. can gain from the increase in their personal vibrations. My theory, which I don't impose on anyone, is that in the past, for example at the time of the Buddha Sakiamuni, people were far closer to the spiritual sphere than ourselves. They lived at a higher frequency level and cases are described where people achieved high spiritual insights not through concentrated meditation but purely on the basis of information from Buddha.

7. Initial Consultation

Autopathic therapy almost entirely obviates the need to find a precisely resonating medicine—the hardest and sometimes insoluble challenge for a practising homeopath. Resonance of the fine-matter creative frequency with the person's own potentised saliva carries the highest degree of probability, with a few possible exceptions. Perhaps the chief of these is a serious error during preparation, carelessness, a major departure from the simple instructions for preparation. The greatest error is if someone else talks, sneezes or coughs during preparation. Small particles of alien saliva will be transferred to the preparation and with them non-material disinformation. Another reason why a person may show no response even two months after using the preparation is that the chronic pathology is so serious and deep-seated that it requires a much longer period of autopathic healing than is common (see the asthma case). Here I should again of course point out that an unknown factor during autopathy is the person's inner, hidden, karmic state. The classical homeopathic therapy may also encounter lasting and serious problems that take years to cure. In my experience, however, autopathic cures of these ailments are generally quicker than their homeopathic equivalent because of the closer resonance.

The golden rule of homeopathy, quoted by the classic homeopaths in capital letters, also applies to autopathy: WATCH AND WAIT for the case's development.

Monitoring the patient's specific development after administering the preparation is an important skill. Periodic expert consultation between the patient and the practitioner is usually necessary if the cure is to be lasting and profound. This is especially so if people begin with autopathy when they are suffering from long-term and deep-seated ailments that require much time before they show clear signs of improvement or ultimately a cure. It cannot generally be expected that the single use of a medium potency preparation will positively affect a person for the whole of their life. That is why it is important to know when and in what potency to produce and use a new preparation. The point at which it is used also has to be decided accurately according to the patient's development. In some cases this may not be for months or even years. In autopathic treatment, our focus shifts to monitoring the case correctly in order to be able to intervene with another autopathic preparation at the right time and in the right dilution.

Taking the case

The future course of treatment relies heavily on the recording of the initial condition before treatment begins.

We record the case on paper or in a computer. It is a good idea at the first meeting to give each patient a diary, which they should keep and bring to each follow-up. It is up to us to teach them how to keep the diary. After taking the preparation the patient should make concise notes of any significant changes in their condition. Generally, the entries will only be on an occasional basis, perhaps once a week, sometimes more often and sometimes with intervals of several months. It doesn't mean that the patient has to constantly monitor himself. On the contrary, only if something out of the ordinary occurs, for example pain, or the disappearance of pain, should the patient make an entry.

The autopathic approach can proceed without a conventional diagnosis of the illness. Of far greater importance for us, indeed of definitive importance, is what the patient tells us about his subjective reactions, his feelings and impressions. In this respect we have to realise two things. First, this is a centuries-old system of homeopathic diagnosis and monitoring of the patient. Conventional diagnoses are too general and don't address the individual character of each case. Second, health is primarily a subjective value. This is the World Health Organisation's definition: "Health is a state of complete physical, mental and social well-being and not merely the absence of disease or infirmity."

For us, what is essential is our desire to revitalise the person's individual fine-matter frequency. We recognise the development of the individual non-material centre, however, by the way it manifests itself in mind and body. That is why, although we do not specifically cure the illness but the inner human organizational system, we notice a psychological and physical development in the individual's health. Particularly in his subjective feelings and perceptions.

Nevertheless, people generally visit us after long periods of conventional treatment, or while still undergoing such treatment, and because of this they initially like to tell us the names of the illnesses and cite the results of laboratory tests and medical imaging. We obviously take note of these as well. Ongoing tests and medical examinations during treatment can provide us with another indicator of the individual's improvement or warn us of a potential relapse.

Autopathic examinations generally take place in the form of an interview. This may begin with a simple request for information, such as: "What can you tell me about yourself?" Or: "So, what's the matter?" We then let the patient tell us everything that is worrying them, ranging from the physical (illness) to the psychological, or even the social. We don't interrupt and don't ask leading questions that require yes or no answers. We may encourage the speaker with phrases such as: "And then?" or "Is there anything else?" A person never has just one problem, for example eczema. All the cases that I refer to in this book perfectly illustrate this fact, this rule. We usually find a wide variety of problems accompanying the main ailment. Some of them the person may not even be aware of, as they are overshadowed by the chief complaint. About others the patient may not wish to talk, considering them to be "stupid", or having the impression that they are not related to the main problem. Every physical problem is always associated with some dissonance in the psyche. We note down everything that we are told.

Among the psychological characteristics that interest us are fears and aversions. Many adult people are overly afraid of the dark, or of a crowd, or of enclosed places, or of contact with other people; men of women and women of men; they have a terror of tests or of appearing in public etc. Often, nobody around them is aware of this. Sometimes even they themselves are insufficiently aware of their fear, its reality only becoming evident during the consultation. These are all dissonances of the mind and should be improved by the autopathic preparation, often sooner than the physical problem that caused them to consult us in the first place. In the same way we can ask about sleep. We may learn, for example, that the person who has come to be cured of eczema suffers from tormenting nightmares but has never told anybody of them. Or that he often wakes up or has even more serious sleep-related problems: he can't get to sleep or sleeps only three or four hours a night. A practitioner in autopathic therapy should be aware of these things so as to be able at a later stage to decide whether the treatment is progressing according to Hering's Laws, i.e. whether the symptoms are being cured and are departing *from within outward*. Or whether the preparation is wearing off and the deeper-seated central problems that have already been improved or cured by autopathy are returning, which requires that a preparation be administered immediately in order to prevent a deeper return to pathology. Of course we never press the patient and always write down only what they tell us of their own free will.

Let us look at an example of the importance of understanding the whole picture of a patient: The presenting complaint was arthritis, but the patient also suffered from strange and unfounded anxieties. After taking the autopathic preparation these anxieties disappeared, and in their wake the arthritic problems improved. Several months after the preparation the anxieties returned, whereas the significant improvement in the arthritis remained stable. This is a sign that the preparation, in acting "from within outward", has ceased to function and that if we leave the case to its natural course everything else will soon deteriorate as well. If the preparation is administered promptly the deterioration will be quickly halted and progress towards holistic health will be resumed. If we failed to register the end of the response to the preparation until the arthritic problems returned we would lose much time and the patient would have to face unnecessary suffering.

Questions may include the following: Does the patient suffer from undue worries? How does he or she react to solitude and company? How does he or she behave in a conflict of interests and under stress, at work and at home? In all these areas and many others the autopathic preparation will strengthen the personality. If at a later stage there is another sudden or gradual deterioration (this doesn't have to be of the same degree as the initial one), this is a sign either that the preparation should be repeated or that the case should be monitored more closely, and that other follow-ups should be arranged at more frequent intervals. Sometimes the deterioration is merely temporary and caused by external stress, and it clears up when the stress passes. A decline in or cessation of the preparation's effect is usually first manifested in the mental sphere. We have to know the original mental state in order to be able to administer the autopathic preparation over time and to prevent a further deterioration at the physical level.

Psychological problems, which either only illustrate the overall state or are a main reason for treatment, may include: hyperactivity with attention deficit in children, learning disabilities, excessive aggression in children, excessive jealousy of one's siblings, excessive shyness or tearfulness, and so forth. It may be any psychological feature which, in its extreme form, is negative and causes suffering.

General features exist that testify to the state of the organism as a whole. It is useful to know the person's level of energy. Whether he suffers from excessive tiredness or not, or what excessively wearies him. His individual reactions, healthwise and sensory, to heat and cold, indoors, outdoors, at work, on holiday. Reactions to the weather and changes in it. Extreme sensitivity to changes in the weather are always linked to a deterioration in the organism's condition and increased tendency to illness. Just as are sensitivity to the cold and extreme sensitivity to heat and the sun and the temperature in a room or in bed. If after taking the preparation the extreme reactions to the external environment first balance out and then deteriorate again (although not in response to temporary pressure), this may be a sign that a further preparation is required. Even in cases where the basic physical pathology remains improved.

Eliciting the patient's personal history forms an important element of the initial autopathic consultation. We record any deviations from the norm in the patient's development, from birth to the present. This may include a problematic birth, childhood illnesses, accidents, psychological traumas in childhood and puberty, chronic ailments, repeated infections, acute illnesses in adulthood etc. We know that during autopathic treatment certain frequency states may recur which the patient experienced in the past; old and forgotten illnesses may return in a milder and briefer form; old "reverse" symptoms may reappear. The practitioner in autopathic therapy should be able to recognise whether a complaint is in fact the recurrence of an old symptom. Reverse symptoms normally pass relatively quickly.

An example: Ten years ago a person experienced repeated throat aches. After taking the preparation his insomnia and depression passed and for a while he enjoyed improved health.

But then, just before leaving to go skiing, he came down with throat ache, exactly like those he had suffered ten years before. Because the internal symptoms had improved (insomnia, depression) and an old symptom had recurred, it could be expected that the throat ache would pass on its own in a short time due to it being a "reverse symptom". It was a return to the same frequency state of ten years before. The best tactic was thus to wait. The organism can come to terms with an inflammation of the throat relatively quickly. The raised temperature, in this and similar cases of reverse symptoms, usually falls sharply on the second day. The temperature is the organism's defence mechanism when it needs to solve something. Patients usually calm down when you remind them that they experienced the ailment, as is clear to you from their records, some years before, and you explain how it will progress. It is of course entirely the patient's choice whether he takes other medication at his doctor's advice. The final decision of how and by what means a patient is cured is always his own.

Specifying the degree of dilution—potency

A person's history of ailments and illnesses is part of their overall condition. Serious illnesses in the past strongly influence our choice of potency. The rules by which we decide the degree of potency (degree of dilution) are directly derived from homeopathy.

We have, however, another, completely new possibility: to work with finely-graded potencies, for example to go from 40C to a second prescription of 80C, as opposed to homeopathy, where the potencies are graded in large intervals (30C, 200C, 1M). In comparison with homeopathy we also use higher starting potencies in order to get a response (instead of using 5C for old people we use 40C). In the case of people over seventy with very weak vitality and very serious problems we can start with 20C. For normal autopathic practice the scale

of potencies in steps by 40C upwards (40, 80, 120, 160, 200...
etc.) is perfectly sufficient.

Choosing the right potency—the first, single use of the
preparation:
The potencies mentioned below relate to the number of the
bottle's refills and emptyings (a traditional Hahnemann or
Korsakov dilution technique).

When using the Autopathic Bottle for vortex dilution
(a newer and more efficient technique) the 40C potency is created from one litre of water, 80C from two litres, 120C from
three litres, 200C from five litres and so on.

40C—For cases of severe disharmony with serious, long-lasting problems, either current or in the past, and which
have a very low vitality, especially in all people over seventy.

80C—For young and middle-aged patients with very low
vitality and a history of serious, chronic ailments.

120C—For people with medium vitality with a history of serious long-lasting ailments.
For people over sixty with good vitality and who have
experienced only mild problems in the past and at
present.

200C—Medium state of harmony and vitality with no very
serious chronic problems in the past or at present.
For people under sixty. The potency most commonly
used in my practice.

over 200C—For people with a feeling of mental disharmony,
but who have not experienced serious physical ailments.
Attempt to grow mentally (improving concentration,
memory, sharpness, appearance, vitality, mood etc.) or
improve resistance to psychological and physical stress
in relatively healthy people.

If you are not certain which category your case comes under, you should always start with a lower potency.

40C may be used *where there are acute problems,* such as fever, throat ache etc. We can go up to 200C for otherwise relatively healthy people.

There are several reasons why it would be mistaken to recommend a high dilution (potency) in cases that require a lower degree of dilution. One is that we need to retain the space to gradually increase the potency. Too high a potency in certain cases can miss the target.

People who are suffering from very serious, long-term physical pathologies and who at the same time have serious psychological problems should start with a 40C dilution.

Where a second or subsequent preparation is used, in the event of a relapse, we need to substantially increase the potency. Usually we increase the potency to twice the original dilution. For example, from the initial 200C (five litres in flow dilution) to 400C (10 litres), after that to 800C, and so on. Exceptions to this are shown in chapter 9, 'Using the Preparation a Second Time'.

If there is a marked unusual deterioration following the administering of the preparation, or there are significant and persistent symptoms, or the pathology is extremely serious and long-lasting and as a result requires long-term treatment, the patient should also seek conventional medical advice. This applies especially as the therapist or person treating himself can never be certain what is the actual cause of the deterioration at the physical level. Following the use of diluted saliva, improvement may first occur (as in many of my own cases) at the spiritual level and then at the mental and physical level, including in cases of consistent conventional specialist medical care.

Summary of the initial consultation:

1) We make a note of *all* current complaints, large and small and however insignificant, both physical and psychological.

2) We keep notes both of the physical side—illness and ailments—and the psychological side—if there are any such problems.

3) We decide on and recommend a potency—the number of dilutions or litres of water. We give the patient instruction on how to individually produce the preparation (it is also attached to the Autopathic Bottle) and write down the relevant potency.

4) We agree a date for the first follow-up consultation. This usually takes place five weeks after taking the preparation if it is a chronic illness that is being treated. The organism needs to be given time to respond. When treating an acute illness we need to communicate with the patient at his or her request (e.g. after hours or days) until the problems improve or disappear.

5) We assure the patient that we are available on the telephone in the event of any uncertainty or problems on their side.

8. Producing Your Own Autopathic Preparation

At the beginning I describe the dilution or potentising process based on the Korsakov principle. This form of autopathic preparation has also been tested. I used it in the early stages of my autopathic practice. It makes the preparation easily available, any time and anywhere, as it doesn't require any special or professional equipment. Any small, clean vessel is sufficient. This form of preparation is suitable for potencies up to 40C, and by using it people can find out for themselves that autopathy can work. More advanced and more effective means, i.e. Autopathic Bottles, can be used later.

The following instructions have been fine-tuned, partly in response to the questions and comments of those people who have diluted their saliva, in order to eliminate any potential errors that might arise during preparation. Don't worry in the least about not managing the preparation stage. It's very simple. Preparation takes one hour at the most, including clearing up, without any rush. It is no more complicated than making a cup of medicinal tea. It is only necessary at intervals of many months. Don't hurry the process and by the same token don't interrupt it. If you find you have problems, ask someone to help you. Or, alternatively, why not give someone else a hand?

How to dilute the saliva

Preparation is usually conducted by the person who will use it, although this is not a condition. If the preparation is conducted by someone else, this person should wear a scarf or mask across his or her mouth and nose during the entire process, so as to prevent drops of alien saliva affecting the preparation when speaking or sneezing. Rubber gloves are also recommended.

Materials:
1) The smallest (e.g. 10ml used for medicinal drops), new, as yet unused empty glass vessel or receptacle (obtainable for example in a kitchen shop, hardware store or pharmacy etc.). Heat the vessel over a kitchen *gas* cooker from all sides on its outer surface until it is very hot using tongs to avoid burns. Then leave to cool.
2) Bottled still spring water (not sparkling and without a high mineral content or artificial additives), as recommended by an autopathy practitioner or by literature about autopathy. For a potency of 40C, i.e., forty refills/emptyings, you could need approximately 0.5 litres of water for a 10ml glass vessel; the volume of water increases proportionately with the potency and depends mostly on the size of your vessel.
3) Rubber (latex) gloves (can be bought at a chemist's).
4) Normal domestic disinfectant.
5) For a nursing child a new, glass, packaged, clean dropper.

Procedure:
1) Carefully brush your teeth without using toothpaste. Then for approximately two hours do not eat, drink or smoke and do not place anything in your mouth. There should be no trace of cosmetics on your lips. Do not use a cell phone before preparation.
2) If you are producing the preparation for someone else you should wear a scarf or surgical mask across your mouth and nose throughout the entire period of production, so that no microscopic drops of your own saliva transfer (when talking or sneezing etc.) to the preparation. You should wear rubber gloves. For babies you take the saliva (one drop is sufficient) during sleep or just after waking, with a hitherto unused clean glass dropper.

3) Place all the materials within easy reach of the basin, including the chair that you will sit on during preparation. Don't touch the rim of the vessel. Nobody else should be present during preparation.

4) Spit out once and then gather sufficient saliva in your mouth before spitting into the prepared vessel. A few drops are enough.

5) Immediately approach the basin equipped with the small vessel containing the saliva and bottles with water.

6) Pour the water into the vessel containing the saliva. Don't allow the neck of the bottle to touch the neck of the vessel. Pour from a height of approximately 5cm. Fill the vessel up to the top, allowing the water to run over the rim so that it wets the entire circumference of the neck. Immediately empty the contents into the basin. Pour in the water, allowing it to spill over the rim, empty, pour in water ... and so on. The drops sticking to the walls carry the information through each dilution.

7) Place part of the final contents (a few drops are sufficient) of the vessel in your mouth immediately after completing the preparation phase. Don't place anything in your mouth, or eat or drink anything for at least 10 minutes after use.

8) Carefully wipe the basin with domestic disinfectant *no sooner than half an hour after taking the preparation* in order to remove the fine-matter vibrations. Throw away the gloves and the vessel used for dilution.

9) Use once only (once is enough)!

10) Individual development after taking the preparation depends on the state of the person's inner karmic disposition. The process isn't simple, just as life isn't simple.
    It's a good idea to use the services of an expert practitioner (via internet, phone or a personal consultation) particularly on questions of when to repeat or increase

the potency of the preparation and at what degree. Progress is not always straightforward.

11) Keep notes on your physical and emotional state and produce these at follow-ups. Only write down significant changes, along with a note of the date on which they occurred.

12) An autopathic preparation diluted to a fine-matter state acts exclusively on the fine-matter (from a materialist point of view completely non-material) governing spiritual principle present in the person. An improvement in his organisational capacity may then lead to the gradual harmonisation of the person's system at many levels.

The use of highly-diluted saliva is not a substitute for medical care. It can be used also as a complementary or adjunctive method and does not disturb other forms of treatment.

Notes:

The preparation process known as the Korsakov method is straightforward and is often used by large-scale producers of highly-diluted homeopathic preparations, the difference being that these conduct the process in laboratories and by means of electrically powered equipment.

It is important to emphasise the choice of vessel. In order to save water it should be as small as possible. It should never have been used previously and should not be an empty medicine bottle. Just rinsing it (see the whole philosophy of dilution) is not going to help very much. The ideal vessel is a small, unused bottle such as those used for medicinal drops (approx. 10ml), sealed with a screw-type plastic lid. Pharmacies usually have unused samples of these in stock and are happy to sell them. Small, new vessels can also be found in shops that sell glass, domestic or laboratory utensils. The main concern is to ensure that the rim and the inside of the vessel do not bear the imprint of someone's hand from the time of its production, storage or sale. Such a print would carry information about that person's frequency structure and could alter the preparation's qualities. I therefore recommend that the vessel's neck be strongly heated over a normal gas ring on your kitchen cooker. This will burn off the imprint. You can test this for yourself: leave a fingerprint on the vessel and hold it above a flame. The print disappears and the glass is clean again. Heat the vessel from the outside, holding it near the base using tongs. One minute over a naked flame is sufficient. Turn the vessel slowly so that it is exposed to the flame from all sides. A naked gas flame should be used, such as that produced by a good kitchen cooker. No other flame should be used, such as that of a candle or lighter. These would leave traces of soot on the glass and would only contaminate it further. A woman contacted me on the subject of these instructions and complained that she did not have a gas cooker, but one with a ceramic surface. Electric cookers are no good for our purposes. In the end she heated the vessel over someone else's gas cooker and brought it home in a clean, unused plastic bag in order to carry out the dilution. It is also possible to use a small gas camping cooker.

Just as good as a bottle is the smallest type of receptacle for alcohol, which can be obtained in all shops selling glass. If the receptacle has a wide, open neck, making it possible for the shop assistant, for example, to reach inside and leave her fingerprints or small drops of saliva there, the whole of the receptacle should be heated slowly over gas from the outside, including the base, for two to three minutes. It can be held over the flame by means of, for example, a knitting needle (which has also been first heated up) or tongs.

There is a direct relation between the size of the vessel and the amount of water used to produce the relevant potency. If you can only find a larger vessel you will have to buy more water.

For a variety of reasons, glass is the most suitable material for the purpose of homeopathic dilution. Nevertheless, in an emergency, substitutes can be found. For example, if you are unable to find a new, unused vessel and to heat its neck over a naked flame, for instance, while hiking, you could buy a normal plastic bottle of spring water and use its plastic top instead of the vessel for the Korsakov dilution (repeatedly emptying and refilling it). Otherwise the procedure is the same, apart of course from the heating. A man told me that in the past he had had good experiences with this method. He now uses the Autopathic Bottles as a more professional, more efficient and reliable means of production.

Whatever its dimensions, we consider one filling of the vessel to be the 1C potency. Five refills of the vessel make 5C, twenty 20C, forty 40C.

You should overfill the vessel slightly each time so that the water spills over the entire circumference. This is to ensure that the previous potency remaining on the rim is thoroughly rinsed off.

When using the smallest vessel, probably 10ml, to produce the 40C potency one needs approximately half a litre of water. In order to be certain, you should have a larger supply of water in order to compensate for the water lost when overfilling.

If your hand begins to tire before reaching the desired potency you should use the preparation in the potency at which you stop. In practice there is no obvious difference between the effects of a 10C or a 15C potency, or between 30C and 40C. The Korsakov method of preparation can be rather demanding manually, which is a certain disadvantage. It is also slower, but on the other hand, it is usually usable as far as higher potencies (over 40C) are not involved.

In order to even out any complexities and resolve any uncertainties concerning the different types of dilution vessels, and to avoid any contamination or manual over-exertion, I have designed a special instrument for personal preparation. I was inspired by the principle of flux dilutions, which were successfully proven in the nineteenth century by Dr. Fincke of New York. I call it an *"Autopathic Bottle"*.

It's appropriate for the simple and reliable production in the home of all potencies, but is indispensable particularly for potencies over 40C. It has a funnel, a connecting tube to the vortex chamber and a waste tube from which the diluted liquid is drained. It is compact and made from chemically stable laboratory glass. The vortex chamber in the lower section causes the optimal whirling of the liquid at constant pressure and its gradual vortex dilution. The Autopathic Bottle represents a simple means of producing the preparation at the highest quality. Among other reasons, this is because there are no interruptions that might negatively affect the process and also because of the special quality of the vortex which has, according to the ideas of Austrian philosopher Viktor Schauberger, a positive "centripetal" character in the latest model with a spherical vortex chamber.

The "Autopathic Bottle" is produced in a glass-works under special conditions according to rules established by the author. It is sufficient to follow the enclosed instructions, remove the Autopathic Bottle from the plastic bag, spit into the funnel, pour through a litre of water or more and the job is done. From one litre of water you can expect to produce a 40C potency in approximately twenty four seconds, 80C from two litres and so on. If you place it under a current of water flowing from the mains water supply through an ordinary kitchen carbon filter it will produce 100C every minute. 1000C (1M) can be achieved in ten minutes, 10,000C (10M) in 1 hour 40 minutes. Any clean drinking water without chemical additives can be used, for instance water from a well, in this case without a filter. Following this procedure you can allow the water to flow over the upper part of the funnel. Treatment is not usually begun with a high potency over 1M, it is commonly reached over a period of time. I currently have several cases on potencies exceeding 1M, as well as cases progressing excellently on 6M and even 10M, and some practitioners have informed me that they are already using 10M and higher.

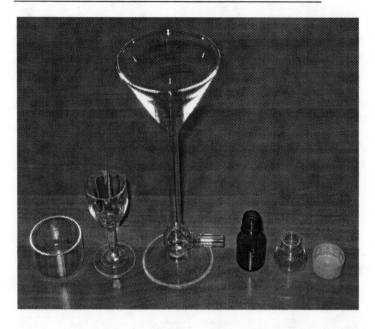

*Various types of vessels and receptacles suitable for the production
of an autopathic preparation, including the Autopathic Bottle
in the middle.*

A person who attended the Homeopathic Academy courses
has even achieved a potency of 50M with the Autopathic Bottle.

The Autopathic Bottle is accompanied by detailed but
straightforward instructions on its use. All the cases described
in this book, and in recent years also all of my "autopathic"
cases, have involved the use of the Autopathic Bottle. I found
the vortex dilution the most efficient in comparison with
other methods of preparation. Moreover all my cases which
I began with the Korsakov method were successfully continued, or cure was completed, with an Autopathic Bottle. The
positive reaction achieved after a single use of the Autopathic
Bottle always lasted for more than three months, even at lower
potencies produced from just one litre of water. In some cases

/117

they lasted for more than two years. The Autopathic Bottle is designed to be used only once in order to avoid the possibility of cross contamination from the memory of the glass, which can retain the previous potency even after the removal of the drops. The production of homeopathic remedies has shown that new glass should always be used in the preparation of new potencies, for the Korsakov method as well as for the vortex flux method. Mixing the two potencies can nullify the preparation's effectiveness, especially if the vibrations of two different people are mixed.

It is important that the production of the preparation from the original spit, through the dilution process and on to its use, is continual, *without major interruptions*—this is easily achieved with the Autopathic Bottle. The vibrational structure of the potentised preparation might alter if left for an extended period of time, for example, for several minutes. If the interruption is even longer, the preparation will completely lose its effectiveness. This was the experience of one of the people who visited me, and he later found that it really does work if the process is without interruption.

The following instructions for use are enclosed in every box with the Autopathic Bottle.

Autopathic Bottle
User guide

Read carefully before producing the preparation.
The preparation is usually produced by the person who will use it, although this is not necessary.

Purpose: "The Autopathic Bottle" is designed for the vortex dilution of a person's own saliva into the fine-matter level. The product of dilution is used exclusively by the same person that provided the saliva.

Philosophy: Through resonance, the product of high dilution acts positively on the fine-matter (from a materialistic point of view immaterial) spiritual frequency organising principle, which can improve its function and in the longer term gradually return harmony to the whole system in a person at all levels. The action is always dependent on the internal state of the individual.

What you need:
1) An Autopathic Bottle made of laboratory chemically stable glass.
2) Ordinary clean bottled spring water (not sparkling and without a high mineral content or artificial additives), in quantity as recommended by an autopathy practitioner or by literature about autopathy.
3) Normal household disinfectant.
4) For babies, a previously unused packaged clean dropper.

Production time including cleaning up approx. 1 hour.

Procedure:

1) Carefully brush your teeth without using toothpaste and for approximately two hours do not eat, drink or smoke, and do not place anything in your mouth. There should be no trace of cosmetics on your lips. Do not use a cell phone before preparation. If you are producing the preparation for someone else you should wear a scarf or surgical mask across your mouth and nose throughout the entire period of production so that no microscopic drops of your own saliva transfer (when talking or sneezing etc.) to the preparation. For babies you take the saliva (one drop is sufficient) during sleep or just after waking, with a hitherto unused clean glass dropper.

2) Unpack the bottle and place it beside the basin or at the base of the sink with the lower drainage pipe pointing towards the plughole. Do not touch the inside of the funnel. No other person should be present during the operation.

3) First spit out, then gather up sufficient saliva in your mouth and spit into the middle of the funnel. Wash the saliva down into the bottom of the bottle using water.

4) Immediately pour the recommended volume of water into the funnel. Do not interrupt the procedure. Do not touch the funnel with the bottle neck, but pour from a height of about 5cm. Ideally (although this is not a necessity), the water should form a surface in the funnel. Overfilling the funnel is not a problem.

5) Immediately after that raise the bottle and through the lower pipe pour the remaining contents of the vortex chamber into your mouth. A few drops are enough. Pause a moment before swallowing. Do not eat or drink for another ten minutes.

6) Transfer the bottle to a plastic bag which you have previously prepared and then it throw away. Make sure

the diluted substance does not drip around the basin. Carefully wipe the basin after about half an hour (*never immediately after use!*) using a normal household disinfectant in order to remove the fine-matter vibration of the highly-diluted substance.

7) The Autopathic Bottle is intended to be used only once. It should never be used at a later time for another person. This would result in the mixing of the fine-matter vibrations of the two persons, so-called "cross-contamination" and the preparation would no longer be effective. It is known from the production of homeopathic dilutions that a "memory of the glass" exists which is able to retain fine-matter information, even if the previous liquid has been removed by whatever means. A new bottle must always be used for another person. A new bottle must also always be used when repeating an autopathic preparation for the same person (this captures the current state, which is different from the previous one). *One litre of water produces a dilution of approx. 40C.*

8) A preparation produced in this way can tune the activity of the non-material spiritual organising system over a long period of time, months or longer, and **is only taken once** (once is enough!). The process is usually repeated after a period in excess of three months. Where there are grounds to repeat the process (see the literature), increase the volume of water.

9) It is preferable to ask the advice of an informed practitioner who can recommend, for example, the degree of dilution of the saliva and who can also advise you, according to your development, on when and to what potency the next dose should be diluted, and whether another autopathic intervention in the spiritual organising system is or is not appropriate. Long-term development following the use of the preparation is not nec-

essarily straightforward and is an individual matter according to the person's inner, hidden (karmic) condition. It is a good idea to go for regular follow-ups. You can draw inspiration from the book *Autopathy: A Homeopathic Journey to Harmony* by Jiri Cehovsky, which deals in detail with experiences and philosophy associated with this method.

10) Keep a record of your condition in a special book. Only record conspicious changes in your development and how you feel, making a note of the date on each occasion.

11) The use of highly-diluted saliva is not a substitute for medical care. It can also be used as a complementary or reinforcing method and it does not disturb other forms of treatment.

Produced in the Czech Republic. The Autopathic Bottle is protected as a European Registered Community Design. It complies with the terms of the Decree of the Czech Ministry of Health 38/2001 Coll., falls under the category of products "used in relation with foodstuffs" and the product is not intended to diagnose, treat, cure or prevent any disease. Highly diluted saliva (beyond the Avogadro limit) can harmonise the fine-matter spiritual organising system, which Samuel Hahnemann called the "dynamis".

The method of *personal autopathic preparation* described above offers possibilities that have never previously been available:

- For the first time in history it offers everyone the possibility, through its simplicity and accessibility, of producing an autopathic preparation of their own highly potentised saliva at home, easily, reliably and according to a standard procedure.

- In following this procedure the saliva is placed in a dilution vessel as it is, *entirely fresh*, and it can immediately be potentised using clean water in its original vibrational structure, i.e., before its structure begins to change. The change in structure takes a matter of minutes. Water is the only known substance in nature that does not pass on any of its own specific information (unlike sugar or alcoholic spirit, for example, used traditionally in homeopathy) to the preparation and subsequently the organism, and which does not have any homeopathic effect of its own. It is quite simply the perfect carrier.

- To this feature you can now add the unprecedented possibility of using the potentised preparation immediately after its production, unmixed with another homeopathically active substance (alcoholic spirit, sugar) and not exposed to any of the long-term effects of the various types of radiation that exist in our civilisation (radio waves, electro-smog etc.) and which are more intense during transport etc. The patient has for the first time the possibility to use the potentised frequency pattern in its completely *unaltered, original form.*

- The vortex preparation in the Autopathic Bottle is far quicker than other methods, capable of achieving high potencies in minutes. This gives rise to another advantage: at the time of using the preparation, the organism's vibrational state, which is constantly changing, is still practically the same as it was when the saliva was removed. The resonance is therefore stronger than was ever possible before.

- For the first time, you can produce the preparation in almost any circumstances, whenever the need arises.

- The autopathic method provides the hitherto entirely unknown possibility of a sort of *gradual multiplication of the preparation's effect.* Through the preparation we improve the frequency of the organism as a whole,

return it in stages to a state of better health, and, from the basis of this healthier organism, we can then create new preparations which strengthen the non-material creative sphere.
- Moreover, in special cases we can increase the potency only gently and slowly, for example by 40C, and not in large steps.

The preparation is generally produced (with the exception of children and the physically disabled) by the person who is to take it. This eliminates the possibility that the material will be contaminated and thus debased, for example by drops of saliva or phlegm from another person producing the preparation (this factor has not been sufficiently taken into account in the preparation of homeopathic medicines). If a parent produces the preparation for a child, he or she should always use a mask covering the nose and mouth. The act of talking, sneezing and so on would, through contamination by droplets, pass foreign information into the preparation, distorting the preparation's effect. I have seen preparations fail for precisely this reason. When a mask was used to produce a new preparation, it functioned properly.

My latest discovery: During the preparation in the Autopathic Bottle you can use an *ascending scale* of potencies. Thus the organism is tuned better and more effectively.

The preparation is done exactly according to the user guide with only one exception: *Once every minute or once after every litre of water we put a finger into the flow of water, running from the waste tube, and lick it. If we prepare it for somebody else one uses a clean teaspoon instead of a finger.*

This method also enables us to reach a potency of the preparation that is as near as possible to the individual fine matter level where the disturbance which hinders the flow of vital force arises. Everybody has their individual optimum potency, which is unknown to us.

The preparation is intended to be used only once. After its use, the long, gradual harmonization of the entire organism can begin.

It is always useful to point out that autopathy is not a therapy in the sense of materialistic science, nor does it claim the reduction or elimination of illness as its primary goal. The preparation solely and exclusively operates on a person's spiritual sphere, which in some terminologies is called the soul, in others the fine-matter body, elsewhere the *dynamis* or astral body and so on. It acts in a sphere which, from a social point of view, does not fall under the terms of "health care" but spirituality, faith in higher principles superior to the material and mundane sensory dimension of our existence. The preparation acts in that sphere in each of us through which, according to Swedenborg, we touch heaven. It doesn't directly affect the physical body or the psyche. All positive changes in a person's health and psychological state, all healing, is the harmonising consequence of the improved influence of this spiritual, higher frequency sphere on the whole of our personality. Autopathy is able to positively influence an individual's karmic disposition. Autopathy also only acts to the extent that the individual's karmic disposition allows. The approach to this method is also dependent on karma. If someone finds this philosophy to not be right for him, then he should seek other forms of therapy. His karma will anyway make that decision for him.

9. Using the Preparation a Second Time

This usually follows after a few months. In my own experience I have yet to come across a case in which a second administration was required within a period shorter than three months after a single dose, either with the lowest, 20C potency, or with the higher versions. The longest period is not known, but some of my cases have been on a single dose for about two years and are still improving. I expect that the longer the autopathic therapy is followed, and the more the health of the patient improves, so the intervals between doses will lengthen. The dose should be repeated shortly after a relapse, a deterioration in problems which had improved as a result of the autopathic preparation. I have already touched on this in various sections of this book. A relapse, a reversal to the state before treatment, usually begins in the psyche. The patient might once again experience sleep problems and persistent bad moods for no apparent reason, all at a time when the physical problems are still improving. If, however, the patient suffered no serious psychological problems before beginning therapy we will see the chief problem reappear. We can judge whether the symptoms are acting according to Hering's Laws of Cure or otherwise, for example with eczema, which during therapy receded downwards, from the face to the legs, and now begins to rise back up towards the face. Where symptoms clearly develop *contrary* to Hering's Laws this is a sign that a new dose is required.

An example of relapse from my own experience:

One year in the middle of March a thirty year old woman told me about her life-long health problem: she had had bronchial asthma since the age of eight. Over the previous three years the attacks had gradually worsened and become more frequent. She was taking various anti-asthmatic medications. She now had asthma attacks every four hours and during them had to use an anti-asthmatic inhaler which allowed her to breathe more easily for a few hours. The attacks affected her in such a way that she was unable to breathe properly and this would get worse by degrees until she used the inhaler. When small she had for a time suffered from eczema, which later passed off and gave way to asthma.

This type of development is quite common. To begin with I recommended a constitutional homeopathic remedy. Three days after taking it the asthma worsened and she had to use the inhaler every two to three hours. After two weeks, however, she was suffering attacks (and using the inhaler) at eight-hour intervals, an improvement on the original state. A few weeks later, though, and everything was back to where it had begun, in fact to a point at which the period pains she had formerly suffered from had disappeared. The homeopathic medication had a potency of 200C, and I would normally have expected a longer period of improvement than a little under two months. I advised her to take an *autopathic potency* of saliva at 160C. This was at the beginning of May.

Follow-up two weeks after use: For two days no change, then two days' aggravation in which there were two to three hours between attacks. Now somewhat better. Has a pleasant and cheerful voice whereas before she had always sounded under stress.

A week later and the interval between the attacks had lengthened to eleven hours! At the same time a rash had appeared on her legs similar to one she had had when a small girl. This disappeared after one week. A clear reverse symptom! She had already ceased taking other anti-asthmatic medications with the exception of the inhaler in case of acute attacks. She felt better psychologically. The asthma was no longer worse in the heat, as it was previously. She gave the impression of being satisfied.

In June she was only using the inhaler once a day. She used it at the first sign of an impending attack.

In August there was a slight increase in the frequency of use—to once every eight hours—partly as a result of stress from the floods that had affected her home region. Her good mood had disappeared.

At the September follow-up she told me that over the past few weeks she had been using the inhaler once every five to eight hours.

During August, therefore, the marked improvement in her condition had deteriorated slightly. This suggested a return to the original intensity of the pathology, even if this had yet to manifest itself. A slight relapse was taking place. Four months after the treatment had begun I thus advised her to produce a higher potency. The treatment continued.

A preparation may also be used a second time when the patient has taken a low potency (e.g. 40C) for a long-term, chronic pathology that is also being treated by several other medications and where even after many months no noticeable improvement has been detected. There also always remains the possibility of testing the patient's ability to respond. We do this by doubling the potency. It is possible that only a higher potency will reach the depths in which the dissonance has its origins. Homeopathy also sometimes follows the same approach. We have to bear in mind that so-called "incurable" pathologies lasting many years and worsening over that time may sometimes be highly resistant to therapy and may only respond over months or even years of treatment by potentised preparation. In such cases, progress can be confused and problematic, just as life itself is confused and problematic. Where problems arise it is certainly not advisable to refuse other expert care as appropriate. Autopathy can also be used as a complementary, adjunctive therapy.

There have also been rare cases where the patient has not responded in any way to the preparation. It is possible that in some cases there was an error in the production stage. For example, someone might have spoken to the person producing the preparation over their shoulder. Or there was a delay of several minutes between completing the preparation and its use, or a long interval during production, as a result of which the preparation was spoilt. A preparation that has not been conserved changes its frequency structure very quickly and it should be used immediately after being produced. Maybe the patient used a contaminated water, or a contaminated dropper was used to transfer the saliva. If so, the preparation should be produced again using a new receptacle. In some cases the preparation's effect then becomes apparent after all. The reason for the preparation's lack of effect, apart from deep-seated karmic, and for us imperceptible, causes (a very rare but not impossible case) might be a mistake of this sort during production. On the other hand, an error of this sort is unlikely, given the simplicity of the production process; no-one should be put off producing the preparation out of a fear of making a mistake.

The upper limit for the duration of the effect of a single dose is not yet known. As with the most successful homeopathic medicines, however, this might be years, or a single dose may even prove to be a definitive cure of chronic problems that will never return. A return to health without the need for further treatment is the objective of autopathy. The chief reason for a shorter duration of (e.g. only three months) might be that the dissonance is located more deeply, in the finer, higher frequency sphere, at a level of potency higher than that taken by the patient. We thus find our way to the roots of the pathology by means of a gradual increase in the potency of the preparation. Each dose obviously needs time to develop its possibilities and bear fruit. A reliable indicator that it is time to use a new preparation and increase the potency is when an ailment that has already improved begins to deteriorate again. When monitoring this we should follow Hering's Laws of Cure.

If old problems return and then pass again the best response is to wait. The temporary reappearance of old symptoms is "the only way to recovery" (Kent).

Follow-up consultations

The first thing to record at a follow-up is the patient's current condition. We can elicit this through open-ended questions or simply by getting the patient to talk. "So, how are you?" "What can you tell me?" "So…?" We then allow the person to speak and try to interrupt as little as possible.

The patient might not always appear very enthusiastic at the first follow-up. He or she may, for example (as happened recently with a woman who visited me), complain of a burning sensation in the eyes, a problem that the patient suffered previously and suppressed through eye-drops. In this case she complained how much it bothered her and how dissatisfied she was. Sometimes, in exceptional cases, the reaction might be so extreme that you ask yourself if you have been of any help at all. It is therefore important, after the patient has finished speaking, to look back at the records of the initial consultation and *compare the patient's current state with the original state.* In the case of the dissatisfied woman, this showed that she no longer suffered from headaches, whereas before beginning treatment she had experienced continual headaches for fourteen days and frequent headaches before that. Neither was she suffering pain from a chronic inflammation of the gums. The right joint of the jaw, which was the last ailment she experienced before using the preparation, had also ceased to ache and was much less stiff.

We thus see that the case clearly progressed in keeping with Hering's Laws, with the internal and most recent symptoms being cured first. Old symptoms return only to disappear at a later stage. Only when I reminded the lady that two months previously she had suffered constant pain in her head, jaw and teeth, and that she hadn't mentioned these once in her current complaints, did she actually recall having had these ailments. It was at this point, when she remembered her recent suffering, that she began to express her gratitude and was very happy to acknowledge that the treatment had indeed been very beneficial. This type of assurance, based on precise monitoring, that the therapy is having an effect and is following the right course, is extremely important. It means a great deal for the person undergoing the therapy. If she had accepted the uninformed opinions of those around her, who told her that treatment by means of diluted saliva was nonsense and that in consequence nothing could improve, she might have abandoned the treatment prematurely, believing those who told her that the pains in the head and jaw had passed through some external influence, perhaps as a result of a trip to the mountains or a change in her work routine or some other cause. Until one day the preparation would cease to have any effect, she wouldn't return to autopathy, and wouldn't be able to use it further.

Memory functions in a peculiar way where pain and illness are concerned. We have inside us a mechanism encoded by nature (surely a healthy mechanism) that causes us to forget painful experiences. It is not unusual for us to forget entirely that something caused us pain once it has passed. Once the woman had remembered the suffering that had disappeared so recently she immediately had greater confidence in my prognosis that the burning sensation in her eyes would also soon improve. And in actual fact it did pass very soon afterwards.

It is obviously far more common for a person to provide a more objective account. This is greatly assisted if he records all important changes in his physical and psychological state that do not fall under normal daily fluctuations. Everyone's state changes constantly, but only significant changes should be recorded. Records should be kept in the diary that I mentioned earlier.

After the patient has given his account and we have compared each original symptom or problem separately with the current state, we can ask about progress since taking the preparation or since the previous follow-up, and about any events that may have occurred in that time. In this respect the diary is essential. Let us suppose that during his life the patient's health timeline was as follows: first, in childhood, rashes on the skin; then in puberty a cough and repeated inflammations of the bronchial tubes; after twenty, asthma. After using the preparation the asthma sometimes (perhaps) worsens slightly, then improves and disappears. Yet a cough appears similar to that which he had in puberty. After the cough passes a rash such as the one from childhood persists for some days or weeks. There follows a period of uninterrupted health. But then, however, may appear the sign of relapse, a rash, as our curve illustrates. The person returns to a frequency state that he passed through at an earlier stage of the treatment. At this stage of development his symptoms are going in an inward direction, against Hering's Laws. Whereas previously he entered it from below, he now comes to it from above—he is thus on a downward track and must take the preparation once more and in a higher potency. If he fails to do so, in time the cough will reappear and ultimately the asthma too.

In some cases the relapse can manifest itself first directly in the inner area of man. Sleeplessness, headache, anxiety, symptoms already removed by the treatment, appear again after a longer period of time and persist or return often.

The diary entries thus help us avoid further ill health.

When treating an acute problem, positive changes are generally already apparent at a follow-up day after using the preparation: reduced suffering at a subjective level, better mood and an improvement on the physical level. It is sometimes not easy to decide whether the illness is acute, or if a long-term, chronic problem has suddenly deteriorated, or whether this is a reverse manifestation of an old symptom, etc. The treatment of an acute problem is therefore not always straightforward. Should any doubts arise concerning the patient's progress, we should consider the possibility of expert conventional care.

After curing an acute illness the organism sets out, in response to the initial preparation, on the path to holistic improvement in health, as described above. The result is the elimination of the disposition towards illness, an increase in immunity and so on.

At the follow-up we should remember the tried-and-tested homeopathic axiom WATCH AND WAIT. It is often better to wait and give the organism time. Serious, stubborn and long-term cases of chronic illness require patience. They may respond slowly and in very difficult cases of residual and deep-seated chronic ailments the organism should be given several months to show real signs of improvement (see

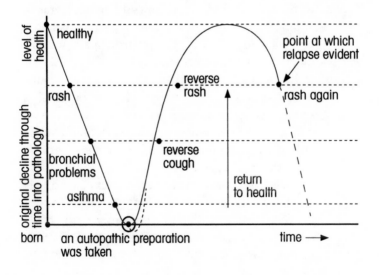

A Refractory Case, page 148). Neither should we forget that people sometimes come to us in very advanced states of serious illness in their vital organs. If their vitality is already very weak the illness cannot be remedied, because the organism is not strong enough. A preparation in a lower potency (40C) can, however, improve their quality of life not only spiritually, but also psychologically and physically.

Summary on follow-ups:
1) Allow the patient to give an account of their current condition.
2) *Individually* compare *each symptom* and problem recorded at the initial consultation with the current state *of that symptom and problem*, i.e. whether it has disappeared, persists, has improved, altered etc.
3) Record progress from the time the patient took the preparation to the present. Establish in general terms how the person feels.
4) Decide whether symptoms are moving "from within outward" or not.
   a) If the case follows Hering's Laws do not recommend another autopathic preparation. Explain that it is necessary to *wait* and that progress may continue long-term in this direction.
   b) If symptoms that had previously improved on the treatment are worse, or psychological or physical symptoms (ailments) return that had already passed during treatment, and these persist, recommend the use of a preparation in a higher potency—usually twice that of the previous preparation.

   If the first potency had a very successful and fully satisfying curative effect for a long period of time (for instance chronic problems were temporarily totally removed), it means that the potency reached the fine-matter level where the cause of the pathology, the defect in the vibrational pattern, was hidden. Then it is recommended to go only slightly higher with the second dose—for instance from 200C to 240C or 280C, or to repeat exactly the same potency.

In cases where the vitality is very weak, in people who are very old (around eighty) or seriously ill, I increased the potency always by 1 litre only. The starting potency was one litre. If there is an indication of a relapse the volume of water used for dilution rises to two litres. If there is another relapse this increases to three litres, then to four, and so on. In cases with a very slow or complicated development you can repeat the same degree of dilution as that used previously.

5) *With the second and following doses it is also always suitable to use the ascending scale of potencies during the preparation (see p124).*

6) If an old symptom (ailment) which the patient experienced some time in the past reappears, check by comparing with the records or by asking questions whether this really is the manifestation of a previous symptom. If it is, and the improvement of the internally located ailments continues, wait and do not use another autopathic preparation for the time being.

On the other hand, if you use the preparation too soon it does no harm except that the progress will be not hastened because it needs its time.

7) Agree a date for the next follow-up, for example two or four months later, if things are progressing in the right way. Remind the person that you are available on the telephone in the event that he or she is uncertain about any aspect of their progress. Telephone and e-mail consultations are a normal part of homeopathy and autopathy.

Part III.
Autopathy in Practice—Case Histories

1. The Importance of Tests

Laboratory tests, CTs (computed tomographies) and other instrument-based approaches, although by no means essential, can also be used together with the patient's subjective feelings and monitoring in order to determine whether a case continues to make progress or not. Their importance lies chiefly in convincing a person who is chronically ill, as well as those around him (relatives etc.), that autopathy is indeed having a positive effect and that this can be proven objectively. Test results may also show a relapse—the point at which the improvement has stopped and it is beneficial to use the preparation once more.

Case: *A young woman*, who some years earlier suffered from an inflamed liver, continues to register poor results in tests on her liver. She has taken conventional medication for two years. Recently, she has experienced hot flushes to her head with occasional feelings of great heat when inside a room. Her right kidney hurts during her period. She has pain, particularly in the right ovary, during her period. A year and a half ago she experienced acute inflammation of the womb and the appendix. She has put on weight since being prescribed steroids. When she gets angry she flies into a rage and her stomach hurts her. She has low blood pressure. She feels unwell when travelling by bus.

I recommend a homeopathic preparation. After two months she reports: The results of the liver tests have worsened and she has begun to suffer headaches. She feels even more tired than before. She often breaks into tears when mentally tired. The hot flushes have not gone away. She has recurring pains in the region of her liver. In other words—a general aggravation. The treatment is basically not working. In this situation it is often necessary in homeopathy to prescribe a variety of carefully-selected remedies and wait to see which one has a therapeutic response. At that time I already had encouraging experience with autopathy and recommended an *autopathic preparation* in the 200C potency prepared in an Autopathic Bottle from 5 litres of water.

Ten days after using the preparation she went for further tests on her liver, which showed a clear improvement. The tiredness passed. Her mental balance returned. The following are the figures from the tests on her liver:

	ALT	AST
shortly before use	2.57 (norm up to 0.73)	1.80 (norm up to to 0.66)
June	1.51	1.24
July	1.47	no data
August	1.61	1.18
September	1.31	0.85
October	1.29	0.94

We can see that her state of health and general mood have improved. Following the use of the preparation, the results of the liver tests, with mild fluctuations, gradually come closer to the upper border of the normal state, registering a significant improvement. She is still not taking conventional medicines.

The reverse symptoms of some former ailments briefly reappeared, including pain in the right ovary, pain around the right kidney and on one occasion in June a headache. She has felt well since the beginning of treatment, unlike previously. The chronic pains in the liver and kidney regions have passed, her energy has returned, and the stomach pains have disappeared. In September she had a cold for a week, only in the mornings after getting up, with sneezing, which was an old symptom (she had previously been treated for an allergy which had manifested itself in the same way). For some months now she has taken no medication. She is more at ease, more balanced, and looks better. She has had no hot flushes for several months. She lost some weight; previously she was unattractively overweight. She seems prettier than before. I have noticed, particularly with women, that they often look much better after a few months of autopathy. This is not merely a superficial observation—they have a healthier expression on their face, better skin quality, are more at ease, and their body language and behaviour are more relaxed. It is an overall impression.

If test results begin to worsen again after having improved with the autopathic preparation, and the deterioration lasts for weeks, this could be a sign that a new preparation in a higher potency is needed.

A quite unexpected development occurred when monitoring the results of tests on *a twenty-seven year old man*. During a chance measurement of his blood pressure he had recently registered 150/105, which is above the norm. When engaged in sustained and heavy exercise (for example cycling quickly uphill) he occasionally felt a pain around the heart and an irregular pulse, the pain always disappearing either during the exercise or after it. The cardiological examination found nothing wrong. Two days after using an autopathic preparation in the 200C potency he measured his blood pressure, which was 139/90, a normal figure. On the third day his blood pressure was 120/80, and continued to remain normal thereafter.

He ceased to experience any unpleasant feeling in the heart region during heavy exercise and no longer had an irregular heartbeat. After a few months he had no complaints. I should point out, however, that this was a man who had been under homeopathic treatment for many years and who had never taken conventional medicines as an adult. His vitality, despite his problems, was very good. In most cases, positive results for people with hypertension (particularly those with a residual illness as well as elderly people and people on medication to reduce blood pressure) take longer to manifest themselves, sometimes up to many months.

2. Chronic Eczema

In 2002, many people came to me asking me to cure their or their children's eczema, although I had not advertised that this was an expertise or special interest of mine. I expect that the television programme I mention elsewhere in this book may have had something to do with it. The programme highlighted the case of a girl whom I had permanently cured of serious atopic eczema. All these people had already tried all available medications before coming to my door. Of course, eczema was never the sole ailment they suffered from. There were always other chronic problems stemming from a greater or lesser general disharmony in the higher creative sphere. Since autopathy "never cures the illness but the whole person" (cf. Hahnemann), and does so according to Hering's Laws (i.e. from within outward), we must always first address the deeper problems and only then can we come to the eczema, which lies at the person's periphery, on his skin.

A slim, thirty year old woman with a reddish face, a graduate of two universities and a keen skier, told me the following story: Atopic eczema from the age of one, when it was at its worst. Her whole life she had treated it with corticosteroids, ointments and pills. The eczema covers her body and her face in red, scarlet stains, with dry skin, flaking and itching, and sometimes she scratches until she bleeds. It is worse from autumn to spring, being very dry during this time. It is always aggravated by stress and anxiety.

Since the age of one she has also suffered from allergies—tests have found her to be allergic to hay, mites, dust and pollen. In addition to eczema, this manifests itself in hay fever during the pollen season.

Once a week she has a bad headache and has to take a pill

for the pain. She is very sensitive to the cold, although she also reacts badly to heated rooms.

A month and a half later she told me the following: Shortly after visiting me she used an autopathic preparation in the 120C potency. The following day the eczema immediately worsened, growing redder and itchier, and she felt as if she had flu. She also had a cold. Right at the beginning she exchanged the steroid cream for a non-medicinal ointment. She kept taking the pills. The eczema remained more or less in its original form (as if she had been using the medicinal ointment), but her headaches improved significantly. She no longer had to take pills to counteract the pain every week. After taking the preparation she didn't once have recourse to tablets. She only had one headache during that month and a half, and even that was mild.

Seven months after taking the preparation: For about three months there was no sign of eczema on her face. It is not hard to imagine how important a change this must have been for the young woman. The eczema had also almost completely disappeared from her neck and chest. It persisted only on her elbows and knees, where it had appeared during the first year of her life. The feelings of nervousness disappeared with the eczema. She no longer suffered from any headaches and, although it was the pollen season, neither had she experienced any allergic reaction! She was very happy and satisfied.

The return of the fine-matter creative principle to its proper function had caused the health problems to retreat from the centre outwards: first the headaches had disappeared, to be followed by the hay fever and finally eczema, disappearing from the head (i.e. from above) downwards.

She prepared in the Autopathic Bottle her last potency of 1.5M (15 minutes under a carbon filter) at the beginning of October 2004 because after a long period of health she had dry skin on her face for two weeks and for two days she suffered from a headache (these were the first signs of a relapse).

At the last follow up in March 2006 she told me that since that time (already for seventeen months) she enjoys perfect health and she can hardly remember the past problems from which she suffered nearly all her life.

The question arises: Was this a cure for headaches, eczema and hay fever? The answer is straightforward: No, not at all. It was a cure for the woman's spiritual, fine-matter principle.

A ten month old baby girl has eczema on her face and all over her body, with the exception of her back. It started during the second month of her life on her eyelids, then affected the face before spreading to the stomach and limbs. The skin is typically red, in some places it is dry and flaky, in others the rash is moist. The eczema itches badly; the girl scratches a lot, even in sleep, and thereby makes the eczema worse. At night she doesn't sleep and she cries. It improves outside in cool weather but is aggravated by bathing. She is highly sensitive to sound: when someone coughs or a dog barks outside she cries. She has a constant need to be held and pacified. She can't bear being alone and can't sleep on her own in a room. Small, malodorous white pustules are forming in her armpits. Her mother tells me she is rather backward in her development: at ten months she still doesn't crawl. I recommend a homeopathic remedy.

Two months after administering the remedy the mother reports to me that the eczema has substantially improved. The child no longer cries at night. The smelly pustules no longer form in the armpits. She walks and is generally much better in her movements.

Another month goes by and her mother tells me: "It's great!" The rash is hardly visible, she no longer scratches her face, but only her hands and legs. It is passing without any further intervention.

One month later the eczema worsened again. The homeopathic remedy was repeated in the same potency and two months later in a higher potency. The eczema again receded, but more slowly than previously. Five months after administering the remedy it lingered in the crooks of the elbows and knees. She still scratched at night. She was given an *autopathic preparation* in the 120C (Autopathic Bottle, 3 litres of water) potency. Five days afterwards she came out in pimples all over her body, which then disappeared over the course of a week. The eczema remained only under the knees. She sometimes scratched in places where the eczema had already disappeared.

Follow-up after half a year: The eczema has completely disappeared. No more scratching. Talks well and is making good progress. Being alone in a room is no longer a source of concern for her.

Another case: Another ten month old girl, with eczema from the age of three months. She scratched terribly, her face was raw, despite being treated with a variety of medicines. Over the previous two months the eczema had improved slightly, although during that period her bronchial tubes had become inflamed. She coughed and wheezed constantly, and her throat was filled with phlegm, which woke her at night. Her mother is asthmatic and is worried because at some point in her life she had experienced a similar chain of symptoms, i.e. eczema followed by chronic inflammation of the bronchial tubes and then asthma. Sometimes the girl's cough would pass, only to return again a week later. In addition, she often vomited and had suffered accordingly for a long time.

The mother gave the child an *autopathic preparation* in the 200C (Autopathic Bottle, 5 litres of water) potency.

Follow-up after one month: The cough has greatly improved and she has entirely stopped vomiting. The eczema (a peripheral problem) has yet to change.

Follow-up after another four months: The child is doing well, doesn't have eczema, doesn't vomit and doesn't cough.

Another case: A baby girl had atopic eczema immediately after being brought home from the maternity hospital. Within a week her whole body was covered. Intensive conventional treatment had no effect. In the fourth month she was brought to my consulting room. She was scratching herself till she bled—at night they had to sew up her sleeves to stop her from scratching. It itched acutely and the child cried all day long. I recommended a homeopathic remedy, although it is difficult to prescribe for babies as their personality features are insufficiently developed to provide an accurate prescription. You have to try a variety of remedies.

Follow-up after one month: Nothing has changed and now the child has stopped sleeping at night. She cries the whole night through—she croaks and wheezes and scratches.

Follow-up after two months: The child still sleeps very badly, and at times doesn't sleep at all. The eczema fluctuates from very bad to better, but with no relief. She scratches at night. I recommended a 40C *autopathic preparation* (Autopathic Bottle, 1 litre of water).

Follow-up after three months: On the second day after administering the preparation the eczema visibly worsened. The child, however, was obviously more cheerful. The next night she slept far better. After one week she slept the entire night, which had never happened before. Her mother said that over the past few months she had slept only half an hour during the day and half an hour at night, and the rest of the time she cried. Three months later the eczema had also improved greatly. She was happy and active.

Follow-up after five months: No rash whatsoever on the face, a little on the neck. Otherwise the rash was only visible at the ends of her hands and legs. Sleeping at night, wakes to drink and then falls asleep again. *Autopathic preparation* at 120C (Autopathic Bottle, 3 litres of water).

Follow-up after six months: Irritable after taking the preparation, the eczema returned on the face the following day. This disappeared again the next day. Persists only on the legs. Had a strong cold.

Follow-up after nine months: Face and body clean. A slight reddish spot sometimes appears briefly and then disappears. Sleeps normally.

One final case of eczema: *A girl of seven*, lively and communicative. Eczema under her knees and in the crooks of her elbows, around the neck. Itched. If someone caressed her she would immediately start to scratch. She had had the condition from the sixth week of life. Her parents only used herbal therapy and acupressure. This had once helped, but no longer. The girl was friendly and very sympathetic, overly sensitive. She often cried. They had discovered several allergies: she had suffocated after eating a poppy-seed cake, and had broken out in a rash after chocolate. She lived in the country. She was also allergic to dogs and horses. After she stroked a dog she came out in a rash and her face swelled up. She was very fond of animals. *Autopathic preparation at 120C* (Autopathic Bottle, 3 litres of water).

Follow-up after one month: Her face reddened slightly after the preparation and stayed that way until evening. After four days the eczema on her legs worsened for a couple of days. Some marks appeared after that, but one month later the eczema had improved enormously. She cried far less than before, as her watchful father had noted.

Follow-up after four months: Until recently, through the summer, she had been free of any problems whatsoever. Her condition had previously always been aggravated during summer. She no longer had a reaction to dogs. Now, though, the eczema had reappeared in the crook of her elbow. My advice was to wait. I considered the mild return of eczema at a time when her condition was otherwise marked by improvements in her psyche and her allergies to be a manifestation of the six year old symptom in accordance with Hering's Law of *from within outward.* In other words, while internal matters improve the surface can still worsen until the organism is entirely healed.

Follow-up after six months: The follow-up did not take place. The mother called to say that they didn't need to come as her daughter no longer had any problems to discuss.

3. A Refractory Case

It sometimes happens that a problem is very deeply entrenched in the organism's history, a factor that causes major structural changes in the organs affected. Initial follow-ups may suggest that the remedy is not working, or is only having a very limited effect. The problems persist for an uncommonly long time. The organism first has to put in order the deeper problems—and we are unable to recognise these because they are located in karma, in the spiritual sphere, or sometimes deep in the psyche. If this is the case the best thing is to wait.

A slim, twenty-three year old man, tall and of sporting build, with asthma. The asthma attacks, of allergic origin, began at the age of five. To begin with they were only seasonal, in spring, and linked to hay fever. Later, they were present throughout the year. The asthma attacks are somewhat improved by the medication that he uses on a daily basis; he currently takes three types of tablet and uses an inhaler for acute attacks. For the last five years the official diagnosis has been bronchial asthma, a condition that his doctors consider to be incurable. A further problem is the nervousness linked to anticipation, the fear he has about every arrangement—meetings, tests etc. It is also a source of anxiety for him that he has problems making relationships and he doesn't have a girlfriend. He smokes a little—two a day, but at weekends up to a packet a day. He is a technician and works very hard. He suffers from flu, which on average he has three times a year and which is accompanied by fevers. The day after his flu inoculation he contracted a proper bout of flu and had to stay in bed for a few days. He continued to catch flu as frequently as before. Recently he has also begun to have problems sleeping. He finds it difficult to fall asleep, problems from work whirl around his head. When he does manage to fall asleep after an hour or more he wakes at four and can't sleep for a further two hours. Then he has to get up for work.

I recommended a homeopathic remedy. After taking this his sleep improved for four months and with it his state of mind. He said that he was better able to cope with stressful situations. The asthma, however, continued essentially unchanged. The attacks usually came after getting into bed and in the night, but also during the day. He stopped taking the medication in the form of tablets and only took the inhaler for acute attacks. He began to smoke more heavily.

Half a year after his first visit he told me that he was living with a girlfriend, and that his self-confidence had improved. The asthma was about the same as before. He slept well.

The homeopathic remedy, administered a second time in a higher potency, resulted in a short-term improvement in the asthma; a year later, however, he was using the inhaler to counteract the asthma attacks on a nightly basis after going to bed. He had also been suffering from back pain for some time.

A year and a half after treatment began I recommended that he take *autopathic preparation* 400C (Autopathic Bottle, ten litres of water). I chose the higher potency because I considered the young man's vitality to be very good, the problems to be relatively mild (his asthma was not life-threatening) and the problem's roots to be very deep in the past. In consequence, a long-acting potency was required.

Follow-up three months after using the preparation: The asthma had worsened slightly; he had to use the inhaler not only before sleeping but also several times a night. Shortly after using the preparation he had also had asthma attacks several times during the day (aggravation following use that in fact foreshadowed an improvement in the future). The attacks during the day passed after one week.

Follow-up five months after use: His first words were: "I'm better." He falls asleep properly, sleeps seven hours and isn't tired during the day. Previously he had a greater need for sleep. His back no longer hurts him. Recently, he had suffered no asthma attacks whatsoever and was off medication. Throughout the entire two years of treatment he had not once caught flu. He smokes two to twenty cigarettes a day, as before.

4. Chronic Inflammation of the Intestines

A man shortly before retirement. He came to me because he was suffering from anxiety attacks, during which he would sweat, had problems breathing and was not capable of doing anything. He was frightened of people. In addition, over the last few months he had been experiencing problems with his digestive system. He had a pain in the left part of his stomach, bad flatulence, irritable bowels and often a watery stool with blood. He was deeply worried about cancer as his father had died of bowel cancer.

Following homeopathic treatment he had experienced a marked improvement in all his symptoms for two years, although there always remained the tendency to relapse back into the old problems. Improvements, though they often lasted for many months, were temporary and never attained the intensity of a complete cure. Blood did not reappear in his stool. After more than two years of treatment he told me that his stomach had again begun to hurt, it bubbled, he had more liquid stools, gas, anxiety, less energy. He was losing weight for no apparent reason. The homeopathic remedy was no longer working. Since the core of the problems was in the psyche— anxiety, the feeling of his life being out of control etc., I recommended an *autopathic preparation* with the high potency of 400C (ten litres in an Autopathic Bottle).

He reported back after a month and a half: The stomach problems had quickly disappeared. He had suffered depression for a few days, but now he had no anxiety and was not fearful.

Two months later I received a note from him informing me that his feeling of health had strengthened still further. He is a trained homeopath who previously had had his doubts about autopathy. He now says his doubts have been dispelled.

5. Advanced Age

An eighty-two year old lady with a lifelong interest in spirituality and alternative therapies. She had a number of serious illnesses: diabetes, ischaemic heart disease, pains in the gall-bladder. She suffered from very bad flatulence and poor digestion, felt a heavy weight in her stomach, like a stone. Constant pain and cramps in her legs, for which she used mint tea. Hot flushes, which caused her many worries, up to four times a day. All at once she would redden and start to sweat profusely. She suffered from low blood pressure; the last time it had been 120/60 and it was sometimes even lower. She felt tired. I recommended an *autopathic preparation* in the 20C potency (only ½ litre in an Autopathic Bottle) and we agreed that she would come back for a follow-up after five weeks. When she arrived, however, she had only been under the preparation's effects for eleven days, as for a long time she had put off preparing it. She told me that nothing much had changed. This is not uncommon. In these cases, the resulting interview almost always unfolds as described here.

I looked at my notes on the initial state of her condition and asked "How are the pains in your legs and the cramps?" Answer: "Much better than before using the preparation." Question: "And what about the hot flushes?" Answer: "Far less frequent, perhaps a quarter their previous rate." Question: "What about the sensation of having a stone in your stomach?" Answer: "The poor digestion and feeling of heaviness in the stomach is much better." Question: "What about your blood pressure?" Answer: "Yesterday I had 130/60" (improvement). Question: "What about your tiredness?" Answer: "Much better. Yesterday I didn't even feel tired." Question: "What about the flatulence?" Answer: "I don't have any."

Follow-up three months later: Gives the impression of being in good mental and physical condition. All improvements had intensified further. Continues, as before, to take a variety of medications recommended to her by doctors over many years.

Another case of an eighty-two year old woman: She has been on insulin for twenty years, takes medication for her heart (she suffered a heart attack twenty years before), for her sleep and for many other problems. She conscientiously visits conventional doctors and has also had homeopathic treatment for ten years. Before beginning homeopathic treatment she used to spend time in hospital every year with some form of serious illness. Since beginning homeopathic treatment she has only once been in hospital. Recently, she had complained that she was losing energy, and was unable to fall asleep at night even after taking a sleeping pill. During the day she consequently felt very tired and drowsy. I recommended that she produce an *autopathic preparation* of 40C (Autopathic Bottle, 1 litre). After fourteen days she was visibly more animated, smiling often. She said that she now frequently fell asleep without the aid of a pill (very unusual) and slept well. Not tired during the day. After another month she showed further signs of improvement. She said that she was having her flat painted, something that she had put off before, considering that it was no longer worth it.

6. Lorry Driver

A robust man of around fifty. Has pronounced dark circles around his eyes. Feels weak; his wife told me that he had recently told her he would soon die. Immediately after eating he has to defecate and his stool is liquid. Has high blood pressure (180/110) even though he has long taken medication to counter this. His back and legs hurt him. His legs hurt him particularly when driving. He specifies that his veins hurt him. On longer trips he gets cramps in his legs and has to stop, get out and rest. He smokes forty cigarettes a day. I recommended an *autopathic preparation* of 80C (Autopathic Bottle, two litres).

Follow-up after four weeks: Four days after taking the preparation he had a headache for two days. After that everything improved. He no longer feels weak. He no longer has to go the lavatory after eating; his stool is not liquid. His back doesn't hurt him, the pain in his veins has reduced; he no longer has cramp when driving on long journeys. He has only measured his blood pressure once, shortly after using the preparation, and it was lower than previously—160/100. He is very satisfied, the dark circles around his eyes are no longer so marked. He says that he has no problems. Despite this, he came for one further follow-up three months later. The improvement had increased. He had not measured his blood pressure in that time.

7. Sceptic

A man in his fifties. University educated, with a keen and lifelong interest in the esoteric. Had suffered from arthritis for twenty seven years. His big toe had hurt him for twenty five years. The pain could sometimes be quite acute. Over the last year the problems had spread to both hands, his knees and also below the ankle. He was taking anti-inflammatory medication, but this had proved ineffective. He was also trying alternative methods and visiting doctors. The problems, however, persisted and were even getting worse. He had soon to leave for Africa. I recommended an *autopathic preparation* 200C (Autopathic Bottle, five litres).

He telephoned three months later after returning from Africa. He wanted to arrange a meeting to talk about the esoteric, as previously. When I asked him how he was progressing after taking the autopathic preparation, he replied: "Well... I don't know. I haven't had any problems for a while. But I think that's due to the stay in Africa. I had to drink a lot and I sweated a lot, so it was like one big sauna." When I countered that many people had fallen ill in Africa, and that it was possible to be quite sceptical about the health-giving qualities of the local climate for a European, he just chuckled down the phone.

I have noticed that for some people with rigid philosophical or religious views (and I include among them bigoted materialists) it is difficult to accept the fact that autopathy or homeopathy actually works.

Nevertheless, some months later he arrived for a follow-up, asked for another Autopathic Bottle and also brought his wife with him as a new patient.

8. Pain

A pupil at high school. She came in November with a headache. This year it has been a cause of frequent pain. In the last two months the pain has been constant. She has undergone several examinations, including CTs, but the cause and remedy have remained elusive. She also often suffers from stomach ache and every two months has a throat ache with swelling of the tonsils, always accompanied by fatigue and high temperature, because of which she is unable to get out of bed. For several years she has suffered from asthma, for which she takes medication on a daily basis and every other day she also has to use an inhaler against acute attacks. Her asthma is aggravated by trips to the country.

Follow-up in January: The headache passed a week after using the *autopathic preparation* 120C (Autopathic Bottle, three litres) and hasn't reappeared. The stomach ache passed after about a month. We see here the operation of the law "from within outward".

First the head is cured and then the stomach. In December, she had twice had throat ache at fortnightly intervals, with swelling of the tonsils but little pain and no fever or fatigue. On each occasion the throat ache had lasted only four days. Twice she had experienced pain around the wrist area, where it had never previously hurt. The pain was moving out from the centre—the head—to the periphery—the hand. The pain in her wrist only caused her mild discomfort.

I asked if she had talked about her treatment with her fellow pupils or friends. She said that she had and that no-one had made any special remarks about it. All of them accepted autopathy as a completely normal and effective approach. Just one fellow pupil had told her that it was stupid because there was nothing in the water. Young people are very open to new things. In the Academy of Homeopathy, which I run, I have in the last few years noticed a big increase in the number of students between seventeen and thirty.

9. A Common Case

Ian, a nine-year-old boy, has suffered from a persistent cough since an early age. Apart from July and August he coughs the whole year round. He commonly coughs up to ten times a day, and often swallows phlegm. The cough causes him to wake in the night. Sometimes it gets worse, and then he has to lie down and is given antibiotics, which he has received twice this year. The cough is gradually getting worse, and the doctor described the latest crisis as the onset of pneumonia. Recently he was absent from school for three weeks, and now he is coughing again.

His mother says that from the age of six months to three years old he suffered from acute laryngitis with a barking, choking cough. It was sometimes so bad that they had to take him for emergency medical assistance for him to be given an anti-asthma spray. He now uses a spray against the cough, but no longer suffers attacks of asthma. He nevertheless suffers from the cough ten months out of every twelve.

He sometimes has jabbing pains in his back, the shoulder-blades and also in his throat. He suffers nightmares, in which he is pursued by dinosaurs and a magnetic man. He has a birthmark on his back and chest. He bites his nails. He suffers from sore skin around the rectum. His movements are very agitated and he finds it difficult to remain in the same position. He is extremely untidy. In the evening it takes him at least half an hour before he can fall asleep, a problem he has had since a very early age. His parents have to read him children's stories for a long time. During birth he was throttled by the umbilical cord.

Check-up after two months: After administering a single dose of a homeopathic medicine with potency of 200 C the cough subsided the next day and changed into a cold. But one month later it returned, although in a less severe form.

/157

Check-up eight months after taking the homeopathic medicine: The cough was better than it had been previously through the winter, and he only coughed three times a day on average. In May he stopped coughing altogether, and he was still symptom-free at the time of the next check-up in June. He no longer has nightmares.

Check-up 14 months after taking the homeopathic medicine: At the end of summer he had a fever, which was followed by a cough and cold.

A few weeks after visiting me he took an autopathic preparation made from his own saliva and using five litres of water (potency 200C, five litres of water in the Autopathic Bottle). Immediately afterwards his persistent cough improved. A week after taking the autopathic preparation he contracted a fever, just like the one he had had recently (the first reverse symptom is the most recent one). The cough reappeared and he visited a doctor, who said that this time the inflammation was not in the bronchial tubes, as usual, but in the throat (the development described by Hering: from within outwards). The increased temperature passed after three days and his sleeping improved. The cough and cold lasted another week. After one month he was only coughing twice a day at most.

The check-up five months after taking the autopathic preparation (in June) showed that he had passed the remainder of the winter and spring seasons with no recurrence of the cough and without any problems.

Check-up 21 months after taking the autopathic preparation: The child had spent the whole period since the previous check-up, more than one year, including the winter, without a cough or cold, without an acute illness, without back pain, nightmares or sore skin. It was the first year and a half of sound health that he had ever experienced.

10. Treating Animals and Plants

Animals and plants also have a creative basis in the high frequency sphere. This is Swedenborg's claim and it is confirmed by our experience with homeopathic remedies, which act on animals and plants in the same way as they do on people. With animals, unlike people, the possibility of individualisation is relatively limited, and the prescription of the most accurate remedy a problem, which is why potentised preparations from their blood, disease products of illnesses, or urine and saliva, are used more often than for people. I do not have any personal experience in using autopathy with animals (after finishing this first book I did and you will find their cases in my second book: *A Homeopathic Healing with Saliva: Autopathy*).

But I quote from the book by the very experienced veterinarian, Dr. George Macleod, *Veterinary Homeopathy* (C.W. Daniels, 1998): "Autonosodes[5] are commonly used when treating cases that don't respond to therapy, where properly selected remedies do not have the desired effect. In such cases, autonosodes usually bring about noteworthy results."

The book only mentions the autopathic approach very briefly, which is typical for the subject in general.

In the case of plants, the search for a simillimum is obviously even more problematic than it is for animals. That is why we know so little about the work of homeopaths on plants and why no specialist literature on the subject exists. Following the rule whereby you prescribe according to the theory of signatures, I succeeded in finding a homeopathic cure for a walnut tree in our garden that had been damaged by the wind. It had lost a third of its crown following a gale, had begun to decay rapidly, developing large cavities and drying up. Its fruit was

---

[5]   Autonosodes are highly-diluted secretions and discharges from a sick person or animal.

of poor quality, and its leaves stained. I approached it from the following standpoint: The tree's fruit were like molluscs. The soft core is covered by a hard shell. The homeopathic remedy produced from the oyster is *Calcarea carbonica*. The problems of people of this constitutional type are often aggravated by the wind. These are people who like to remain in one place, where they feel at home (like a tree). The walnut tree needs a lot of calcium, which is the same material that the oyster shell is made from. Proceeding from these reflections, I inserted a tablet of *Calcarea carbonica* 30C under the bark in a notch that I carved out with a knife. The tree's decline was arrested, the cavities retracted somewhat and new branches grew in the gaps in the crown. This was about fifteen years ago and the tree is still doing well, having resisted many more gales. If you have a walnut tree, try using *Calcarea carbonica* on it. If you have other trees try autopathy. The best method is to dilute sap according to the instructions outlined in this book, or, alternatively, a leaf that has been ground in a mortar using distilled water and a ceramic pestle. The mortar and pestle should be new and should be strongly heated over a gas flame before use in order to remove any fingerprints. It might even be sufficient to leave a living leaf that is still connected to the plant or flower to soak for two hours in distilled water. Other means of obtaining material for potentising I leave to the imagination of gardeners.

The preparation should be dropped into water, which is then immediately sprinkled over the whole of the plant, but mainly its leafy part. Where several identical plants are unhealthy (e.g. in a bed or forest) the material for autopathic preparation can be taken from just one sick plant.[6]

---

[6]   The Dutch author and agronomist Hans Andeweg writes of positive experiences in the autopathic (auto-isopathic) treatment of plants in his book *In Resonance with Nature* (*In Resonatie met de Natuur*, Kosmos, Utrecht, 2000).

Part IV.
Self-Healing

When following the autopathic approach it is advisable to use the services of an informed practitioner who has completed a course, has a certain amount of experience, knows how cases similar to yours develop and is sensitive to your problems. For more serious ailments especially you may need someone whose advice you can rely on at critical moments. It is possible that you don't know such a person and can't get hold of one. Or you may not want to look for one and would like to try it for yourself. If so, autopathic self-treatment is certainly appropriate and practical for you. It is accessible and can be used by everyone, today or at the latest tomorrow. Moreover, autopathy does not in any way interfere with other courses of treatment and does not introduce any alien vibrations into the organism. It can also be used entirely naturally as a complement to any form of therapy, as an adjunctive treatment, strengthening your physical and psychological condition etc. The use of traditional medicines does not render autopathy ineffective. Unlike standard medications, autopathy operates in a spiritual realm where it cannot have any competition. It acts at a different, higher level. That is why people who take medication show almost identical progress as those who don't. Conventional medicine generally does not counteract the effects of the autopathic method. Of course, the aim is to improve the state of health to the extent that no medication is needed.

Concise information for self-help work on oneself or others—without the assistance of an expert practitioner and using the Autopathic Bottle.

1) Individually appropriate amount of water for dilution for the first use of the Autopathic Bottle according to the type of personality:

1 litre (40C)

In strongly disharmonised cases with prolonged serious problems either in the present or the past. In cases with a very poor vitality, especially people over sixty.

2 litres (80C)

Young or middle-aged people with poor vitality and long history of persistent serious problems.

3 litres (120C)

People with average vitality with long history of prolonged problems. People over 60 with good vitality and minor current or past problems.

5 litres (200C)

Satisfactory state of harmony and vitality with minor continuous problems in the present or in the past in cases of people younger than 60.

More than 5 litres

People with a feeling of mental disharmony but no present or past serious disorders on the physical level. Relatively healthy people in pursuit of mental growth (improvement of concentration, memory, shrewdness, insight, vitality, mood etc.) or increased resistance against mental and physical stresses.

If in doubt as to which category your case belongs, use a smaller amount.

2) In a diary or notebook briefly write down all the disharmonies, ailments or problems and sensations, both mental and physical, that you currently experience and

can observe. Resist the temptation to provide diagnoses. Each ailment and everything we want to improve in ourselves should go on a separate line. Put the date.

3) Produce and use the preparation according to the user guide included in every container of the Autopathic Bottle, taking into account the recommended amount of water suitable for your state.

4) On a regular basis, note down in the diary any conspicuous changes in the way you feel and how you observe your condition. For example: *7.10.2002—headache in the afternoon.* Or: *10.11.2003—Stomach pain much better.* Or: *3.12.2009—Rash on right hand disappeared. Temperature of 37.7 degrees centigrade, afternoon.* This is the way to keep notes, sometimes only once a month, at other times three times a week, according to whether something has happened or not.

5) After a month and a half return to the original entry at the beginning and read through each ailment separately. Stop at each one and ask yourself:
Do I still have this? Is it exactly the same? Has it changed and if so, how?
Write down the answers under that day's date. If something has improved your confidence will rise. At the beginning it may be just a small change in the psyche— an irrational fear has disappeared, sleep has improved a little etc. We remain aware that in cases of prolonged disharmonies, the process of harmonization is gradual, sometimes lengthy, and not always easy, depending on our inner karmic state. The longer we have had a problem, the longer the healing process will last.

6) Carry out the follow-up described in point 4) every two or four months, or as often as you see fit, although no more than once a month when treating long-term chronic ailments (with the exception of crises etc.). Compare the situation with the previous follow-up and

with the original situation. Also note down what we call "life feeling"—a sense of well-being or its absence, your mood, how you react in stressful conditions etc.

7) If we find that an ailment that has *already been cured* autopathically or has *significantly improved* is now returning again to the pre-treatment state and is tending to persist for days or weeks, produce and use the preparation again, but this time with a larger amount of water (higher potency) than that used in the initial phase. This usually happens not sooner than after three months. If there are no more changes for the better over a considerable period of time (several months), do the same again.

Never throw away the diary/notes. They may come in useful many years later.

The same rules apply when we treat a partner, friend, child etc. Each one must have their own diary.

If uncertain, study literature on autopathy or contact a practitioner.

Part V.
Courses

I started organising courses in autopathy at the beginning of 2003. I have closely monitored the development of a large number of people undergoing autopathic treatment and have learned much in the process. To this I can bring the knowledge and experience of my twenty-two years of homeopathic practice and my lectures at the Homeopathic Academy. I want to share all this with people who intend to act as autopathy practitioners in their families, among friends or professionally in their work as healers or psychologists, physicians etc., as well as with people who are treating themselves.

Analyses of cases from the initial examination and subsequent follow-ups form the core of my lectures. Some of those who sought my advice have agreed to their consultations being video-recorded and allowed their use for teaching purposes. Every case is different, individual, yet in them much can be found of general and common interest that can help us with other cases: The structure of an autopathic interview, how to conduct the follow-ups, when to decide to increase the preparation's potency, the patient's characteristics and qualities that lead us to choose the right potency, mistakes that may occur during the preparation's production, and so on. The subjects are numerous. One of these is the art of explaining how the preparation works and the philosophy associated with this method. If someone knows nothing of this and concentrates solely on the technical side, he will never be cured. This is not because of the "your faith has healed you" approach… but then again, yes it is. In other words, a person who only sees a strange and unusual way of producing the preparation, which he can forget after a short while, is likely to ascribe any positive changes to other "more acceptable", "realistic" and "comprehensible" factors and explanations. When the effect of the first preparation begins to wear off after some months or years, he is unlikely to return to it. A practitioner, on the other hand, monitors dozens or hundreds of cases and is in a true position to see that these in many respects progress in identical ways, and that the use of the preparation was in each case the turnaround point. The practitioner must be someone who is familiar with these things. The work takes place in the higher vibrational creative sphere, which is sometimes called spiritual. It is spiritual consultancy. In order that the practitioner can ascertain what is happening "up there" at the spiritual level in which he wants to operate by means of the resonance, and which he wants to improve or cure, he must first learn to monitor what is going on below, in the region accessible to our senses, in the body and the mind. He is the messenger of good karma. In former times, spirituality and healing were firmly connected. And that is how it is now, albeit rather differently than before, in autopathy.

Participants at courses are able to exchange experiences, to learn and work together. Collective experience reinforces the conviction that autopathy is highly effective and necessary, something indeed for which our own times are ready.

In conclusion, I would like to make a small observation. Astrologists claim that the new millennium should be the age of Aquarius. And it is true that in recent years we have seen that the element of water has begun to play an extraordinary role in our environment. Unprecedented rain and floods have recently entered our lives. As has autopathy, a cure by water, bringing harmony. Water can destroy and it can help, always in harmony with what we ask for through our thoughts and actions.

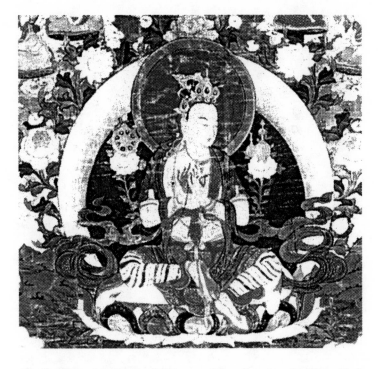

The Buddha of the future, Maitreya, with receptacle called "kundika"
on his left. The receptacle contains pure water which is to heal the
world. Thangka, painting (detail). Tibet, 18th century.
National Gallery, Prague.

Bibliography

Andeweg, H.: *In Resonatie met de Natuur*, Kosmos, Utrecht 2000

Ashin Ottama: *Karma, Rebirth, Samsara*, Dharma Gaia, Prague 1999

Bailey, Philip M.: *Carcinosinum*, 1998

Book of the Kindred Sayings (Samyutta-Nikaya), Pali Text Society, London 1975

British Homeopathic Library, a web site, www.hom-inform. org

British Homeopathic Journal, Faculty of Homeopathy, London

Coats, C.: *Living Energies*, Gateway Books, Bath 1996

Cehovsky, Jiri: *Homeopathy—More Than a Cure*, Alternativa, Prague 1994

Cehovsky, Jiri: *A Homeopathic Healing with Saliva: Autopathy*, Alternativa, Prague 2005

Cehovsky, Jiri: *Speichel der heilende Saft*, Windpferd, Aitrang 2004

Hahnemann, Samuel: *Organon of Medicine*, 6th edition (*Organon der Heilkunst*), translated by Naudé, Kunzli and Pemberton, English edition, Cooper Publishing, Blaine, Washington 1982

Handley, R.: *A Homeopathic Love Story*, North Atlantic Books, Berkeley 1990

Homeopathic software Kent, Alternativa, Medisoft, Prague 1996

Hui Bon Hoa, J., 'Carcinosin: A Clinical and Pathogenetic Study', The British Homoeopathic Journal, pp 189–199, source Reference Works by David Warkentin, KHA, San Rafael 2000

Julian, O.A.: *Materia Medica of the Nosodes*, Jain Publishing, New Delhi 1982

Kent, J. T.: *Lectures on Materia Medica*, Jain Publishers, New Delhi

Kent, J. T.: *Lectures on Homoeopathic Philosophy*, Jain Publishers, New Delhi

Kent, J. T.: *Lesser Writings, Aphorisms and Precepts*, Jain Publishers, New Delhi 1992

Macleod, G., *A Veterinary Materia Medica and Clinical Repertory with a Materia Medica of the Nosodes*, C.W. Daniel, Saffron Walden 1992

Medical Advance, volume XXXII, no. 2, 1894, p. 59, source Reference Works by David Warkentin, KHA, San Rafael 2000

Mistrovská díla asijského umění ze sbírek NG, Prague 2003

Murphy, Robin: *The Medical Repertory*, Hahnemann Academy of North America, 1998

Narada Maha Thera: *The Buddha and His Teachings*, The Buddhist Publication Society, Kandy 1980

Nyanasatta Thera: *Basic Tenets of Buddhism*, Ananda Semage, Rajagiria

Postulka, P.: 'Autopatie', Homeopatie No. 39/2003, p.3, Alternativa, Prague

Superstring Theory, a web site, www http://superstringtheory. com

Swedenborg, Emanuel: *Heaven and Hell*

Swedenborg, Emanuel: *The Intercourse Between the Soul and the Body*

Warkentin, David K.: Reference Works (a homeopathic software programme), articles and references, KHA, San Rafael 2000

Watson, Ian: *A Guide to the Methodologies of Homeopathy*, Cutting Edge Publications, Kendal 1999

Winston, J., *The Faces of Homeopathy*, Great Auk Publishing, Tawa 1999

Contacts

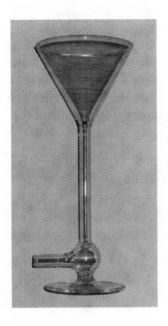

For more information about the method, Autopathic Bottles and their availability, about lectures and seminars:
www.autopathy.info

Alternativa Ltd.
E. Premyslovny 380
156 00 Prague 5
Czech Republic
European Union
info@alternativa.cz

A Homeopathic Healing with Saliva: Autopathy

A further book on the same topic by the same author. New experiences. Thirty new analyses of cured or markedly improved cases of chronic (so-called "incurable") problems as well as a clear and concise "how to" description. A self-help manual. Forthcoming.

Printed in the United States
90528LV00002B/67/A